# 100 No-Equipment Workouts
## Volume 1
## 2017

N. Rey | darebee.com

Printed in the United Kingdom. First Printing, 2016

ISBN 13: 978-1-84481-980-5
ISBN 10: 1-84481-980-9

Warning and Disclaimer
Although every precaution has been taken to verify the accuracy of the information contained herein, the author and publisher assume no responsibility for any errors or omissions. No liability is assumed for damage or injury that may result from the use of information contained within.

# 100 workouts

1. One & One
2. 2-Minute Workout
3. 12-Count Burpee
4. 180 Action
5. 1000 Points
6. Abs Defined
7. Abs of Steel
8. Achilles
9. Aim to Misbehave
10. Airborne
11. Amazon
12. Anchor'd
13. Armor Abs
14. Arms of Steel
15. Bacon
16. Balance
17. Beast
18. Bodyguard
19. Body Hack
20 Borderline
21. Boulder
22. Boxer
23. Boxer HIIT
24. Boy, that escalated
25. Cardio & Core
26. Chisel
27. Close Contact
28. Code of Abs
29. Codex
30. Coffee Break
31. Combat Strength
32. Contender
33. Core Connect
34. Crucible
35. Daily Burn
36. Daily Workout
37. Dash
38. DNA: rewrite
39. Double Up
40. Dynamic Pyramid
41. Eliminator
42. Epic
43. Express
44. Extractor
45. Far Point
46. Five Minute Plank
47. Flash Point
48. Fremen
49. Frost
50. Gamer
51. Gladiator
52. Golem
53. Gravity
54. Grounder
55. Guardian
56. Guardsman
57. Hell's Circuit
58. Hercules
59. Homemade Back
60. Hopper
61. Huntress
62. Infinity
63. Ivy
64. Jacks Pyramid
65. Knee Workout
66. Leg Day
67. Loop
68. Lower Back
69. Make me a Sandwich
70. Mass Blast
71. Master Pack
72. Maximus
73. Movie Night
74. Neck Workout
75. Ninja
76. Odin
77. Office
78. Parkour
79. Park Workout
80. Power 15
81. Pie
82. Pillow Fight
83. Playground
84. Power Up
85. Push, squat, repeat
86. Quicksilver
87. Ranger
88. Rebel
89. Red Warrior
90. Roaster
91. Rogue
92. Run, you clever boy
93. Seated Yoga
94. Shieldmaiden
95. Shifter
96. Silver
97. Sofa Abs
98. Standing Abs
99. Star Master
100. Swan

# Introduction

Bodyweight training may look easy, but if you are not used to it, it's very far from that. It is just as intense as running and it is just as challenging so if you struggle with it at the very beginning, it's perfectly ok – you will get better at it once you start doing it regularly. Do it at your own pace and take longer breaks if you need to.

You can start with a single individual workout from the collection and see how you feel. If you are new to bodyweight training always start any workout on Level I (level of difficulty).

You can pick any number of workouts per week, usually between 3 and 5 and rotate them for maximum results.

Some workouts are more suitable for weight loss and toning up and others are more strength oriented, some do both. To make it easier for you to choose, they have all been labelled according to FOCUS, use it to design a training regimen based on your goal.

High Burn and Strength oriented workouts will help you with your weight, aerobic capacity and muscle tone, some are just more specialized, but it doesn't mean you should exclusively focus on one or the other. Whatever your goal with bodyweight training you'll benefit from doing exercises that produce results in both areas.

This collection has been designed to be completely no-equipment for maximum accessibility so several bodyweight exercises like pull-ups have been excluded. If you want to work on your biceps and back more and you have access to a pull-up bar, have one at home or can use it somewhere else like the nearest playground (monkey bars), you can do wide and close grip pull-ups, 3 sets to failure 2-3 times a week with up to 2 minutes rest in between sets in addition to your training. Alternatively, you can add pull-ups at the beginning or at the end of every set of a Strength Oriented workout.

**All of the routines in this collection are suitable for both men and women, no age restrictions apply.**

# The Manual

Workout posters are read from left to right and contain the following information: grid with exercises (images), number of reps (repetitions) next to each, number of sets for your fitness level (I, II or III) and rest time.

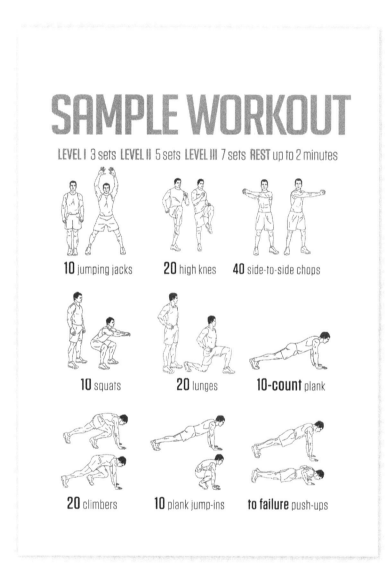

## SAMPLE WORKOUT

**LEVEL I** 3 sets **LEVEL II** 5 sets **LEVEL III** 7 sets **REST** up to 2 minutes

**10** jumping jacks

**20** high knes

**40** side-to-side chops

**10** squats

**20** lunges

**10-count** plank

**20** climbers

**10** plank jump-ins

**to failure** push-ups

**Difficulty Levels:**

Level I: normal
Level II: hard
Level III: advanced

## 1 set

**10 jumping jacks**
**20 high knees** ( 10 each leg )
**40 side-to-side chops** ( 20 each side )
**10 squats**
**20 lunges** ( 10 each leg )
**10-count plank** (hold while counting to 10)
**20 climbers** ( 10 each leg )
**10 plank jump-ins**
**to failure push-ups** ( your maximum )

**Up to 2 minutes rest between sets**

30 seconds, 60 seconds or 2 minutes - it's up to you.

"Reps" stands for repetitions, how many times an exercise is performed. Reps are usually located next to each exercise's name. Number of reps is always a total number for both legs / arms / sides. It's easier to count this way: e.g. if it says 20 climbers, it means that both legs are already counted in - it is 10 reps each leg.

Reps to failure means to muscle failure = your personal maximum, you repeat the move until you can't. It can be anything from one rep to twenty, normally applies to more challenging exercises. The goal is to do as many as you possibly can.

The transition from exercise to exercise is an important part of each circuit (set) - it is often what makes a particular workout more effective. Transitions are carefully worked out to hyperload specific muscle groups more for better results. For example if you see a plank followed by push-ups it means that you start performing push-ups right after you've finished with the plank avoiding dropping your body on the floor in between.

There is no rest between exercises - only after sets, unless specified otherwise. You have to complete the entire set going from one exercise to the next as fast as you can before you can rest.

What does "up to 2 minutes rest" mean: it means you can rest for up to 2 minutes but the sooner you can go again the better. Eventually your recovery time will improve naturally, you won't need all two minutes to recover - and that will also be an indication of your improving fitness.

Recommended rest time:

Level I: 2 minutes or less
Level II: 60 seconds or less
Level III: 30 seconds or less

If you can't do all out push-ups yet on Level I it is perfectly acceptable to do knee push-ups instead. The modification works the same muscles as a full push-up but lowers the load significantly helping you build up on it first. It is also ok to switch to knee push-ups at any point if you can no longer do full push-ups in the following sets.

**Video Exercise Library**
**http://darebee.com/exercises**

The workouts are organized in alphabetical order so you can find the workouts you favor easier and faster.

## 1 One & One

Get up close and personal with your inner being with minute-long workout routines followed by minute-long breaks in between. This is interval training. It primes up your system, helps you burn fat. It will challenge you irrespective of your fitness level as you can simply up the intensity of each rep, in each set, for that special burn.

**Focus: High Burn**

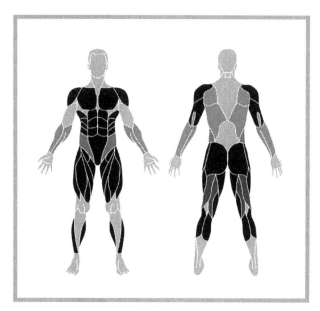

# one & one

DAREBEE WORKOUT © darebee.com

**1 minute** each exercise | **1 minute** rest between each

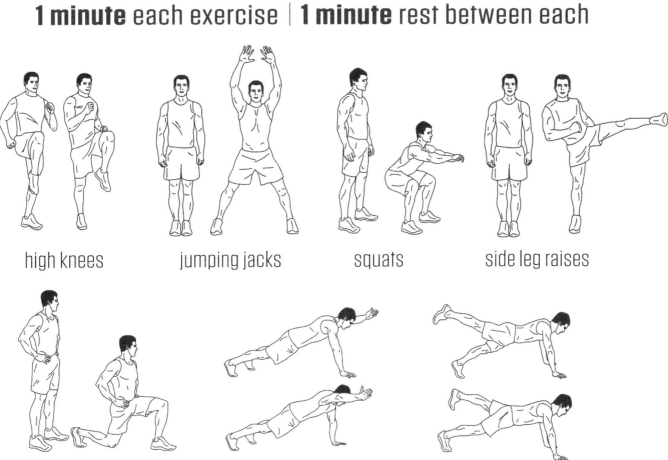

high knees     jumping jacks     squats     side leg raises

lunges     plank arm raises     plank leg raises

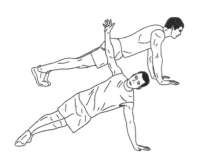
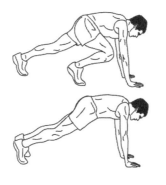
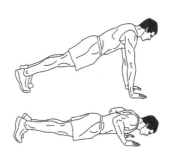

planks with rotations     climbers     push-ups

# 2  2-Minute Workout

No rest for the wicked and this is a truly wicked set of exercises. This is a high intensity workout for the lower body designed to help you achieve explosiveness. Start off at any level you feel comfortable with but do it flat-out each time to reap the benefits.

**Focus: High Burn**

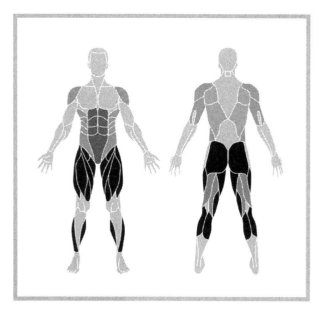

# 2-minute WORKOUT

by DAREBEE © darebee.com

**20 seconds each exercise** | no rest between exercises

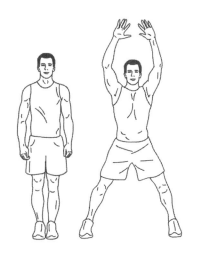

jumping jacks

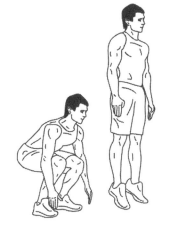

jump squats

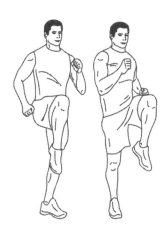

high knees

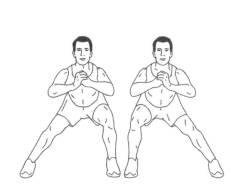

side-to-side lunges

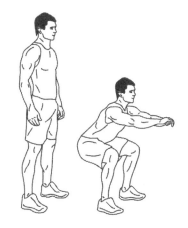

squats

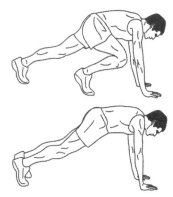

climbers

## 3    12-Count Burpee

One burpee to beat them all. This is a super-set of the classic burpee exercise. The twelve-step program to the perfect burpee set can be practiced anywhere you have a little bit of floor space, making this the perfect exercise routine to have with you when you travel.

**Focus: High Burn**

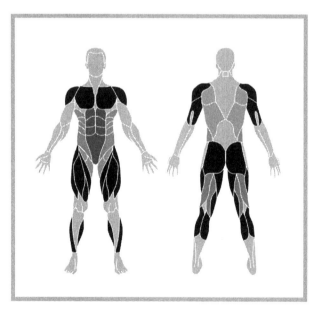

# 12-COUNT
# BURPEE

DAREBEE WORKOUT © darebee.com

**LEVEL I** 10 burpees  **LEVEL II** 20 burpees  **LEVEL III** 30 burpees

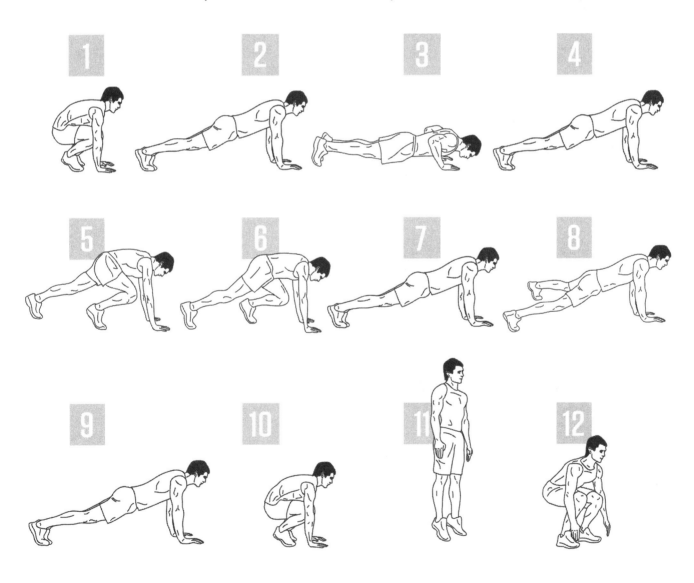

## 4 180 Action

With exercise small changes can produce surprisingly large results. A change of direction each time you floor tap not only provides some variation but it also challenges your body's tendency to fall into an optimized routine that minimizes the energy required to do anything. This makes the exercises physically challenging but there are other, hidden benefits to this: by changing direction each time the exercises become harder from a cognitive recognition perspective. In short they challenge your brain, forcing it to work harder to adapt. Exercise helps achieve significant gains in mental clarity, coordination and even raise IQ points.

**Focus: High Burn**

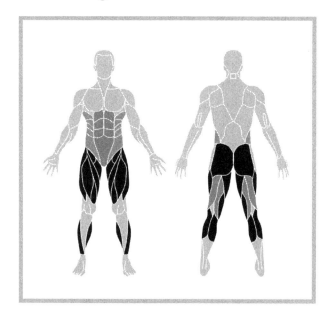

# 180º action

DAREBEE WORKOUT © darebee.com

**LEVEL I** 3 sets  **LEVEL II** 5 sets  **LEVEL III** 7 sets  **REST** up to 2 minutes

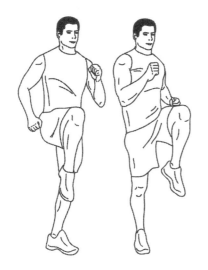

**40** high knees

jump squat

**40** high knees

jump squat

**40** high knees

jump squat

**40** high knees

jump squat

**40** high knees

jump squat

rest

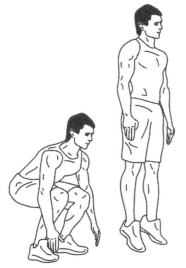

**change direction** after every jump squat
hop up and reverse at 180º facing the other way

## 5    1000 Points

Reward yourself with a point and feel good about what you do with a workout designed to supercharge your body. The 1000 point, total body workout will see you take to the air as well as command the ground.

**Focus: High Burn**

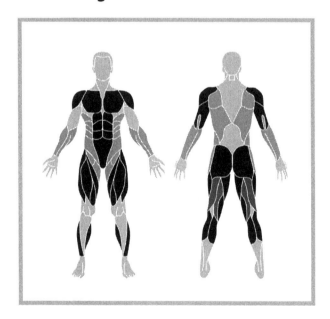

# 1000 POINTS

DAREBEE WORKOUT © darebee.com

throughout the day workout   **each rep = 1 point**

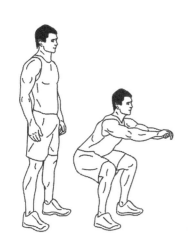

squats

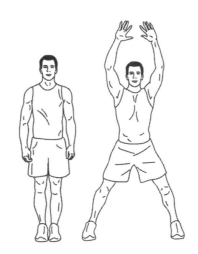

jumping jacks

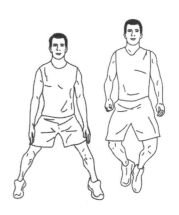

hop heel clicks

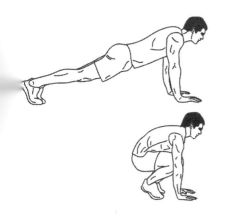

plank jump-ins

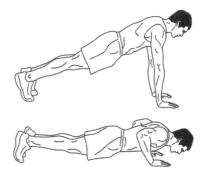

push-ups

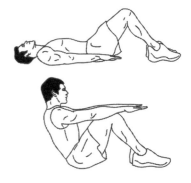

sit-ups

## 6    Abs Defined

Streamline your body, change your posture and add additional power to your every routine with the Abs Defined workout. Not only will you be able to feel the change in the way you walk but you will also see the difference every time you perform any exercise.

**Focus: Abs**

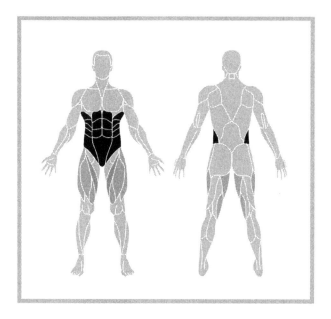

# abs defined

DAREBEE WORKOUT © darebee.com

**LEVEL I** 3 sets **LEVEL II** 4 sets **LEVEL III** 5 sets **REST** up to 2 minutes

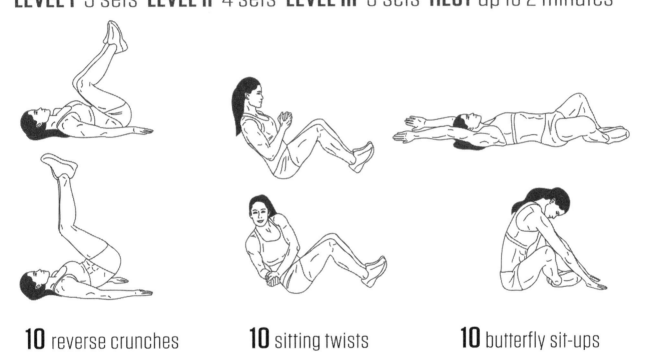

**10** reverse crunches          **10** sitting twists          **10** butterfly sit-ups

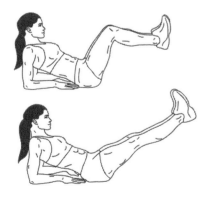
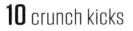
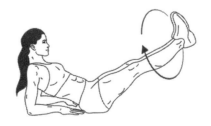
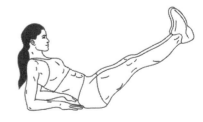

**10** crunch kicks          **10** raised leg circles          **10-count** raised leg hold

# 7 Abs of Steel

Abdominal muscles are body armour. They help protect your vital organs from damage. They keep your body performing at maximum and, when the clothes come off, they make you look terrific. This workout is the anvil where that armour is fashioned.

**Focus: Abs**

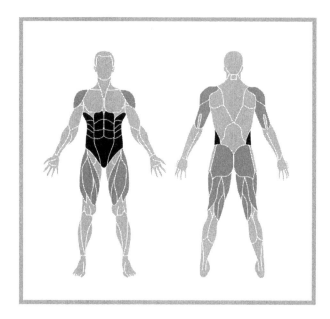

# abs of steel

DAREBEE WORKOUT © darebee.com

**LEVEL I** 3 sets **LEVEL II** 4 sets **LEVEL III** 5 sets **REST** up to 2 minutes

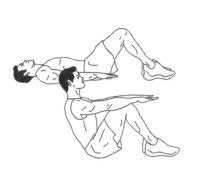

**10** sit-ups

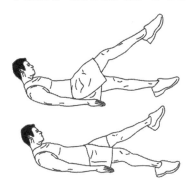

**10** flutter kicks

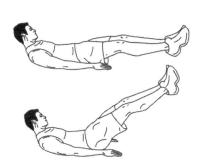

**10** leg raises

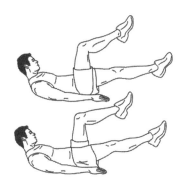

**10** air bike crunches

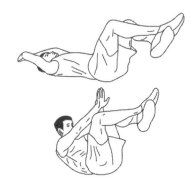

**10** knee crunches

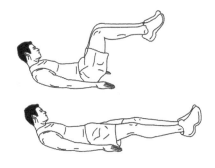

**10** crunch kicks

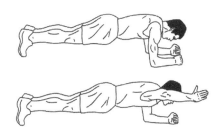

**10** plank arm raises

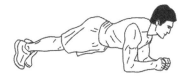

**30sec** elbow plank

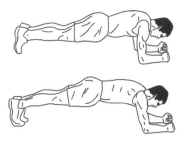

**10** body saw

## 8 Achilles

The body is made up of two basic sections: upper body and lower body. Physical power emerges by forging a better synchronized connection of the two. The Achilles workout aims to help you do just that through a series of routines that will make you feel you're working hard.

**Focus: High Burn**

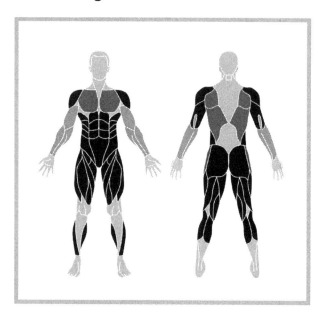

# ACHILLES

DAREBEE WORKOUT © darebee.com

**LEVEL I** 3 sets  **LEVEL II** 5 sets  **LEVEL III** 7 sets  **REST** up to 2 minutes

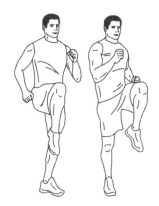

**20** high knees

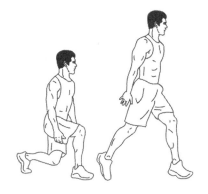

**20** jumping lunges

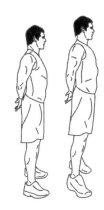

**20** calf raises

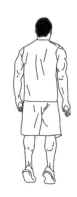

**20-count** calf raise hold

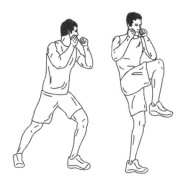

**20combos**  knee strike + elbow strike

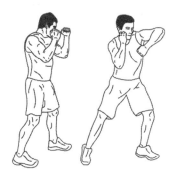

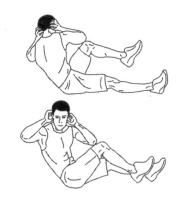

**10** knee-to-elbow crunches

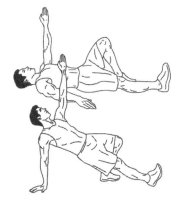

**10** get-ups

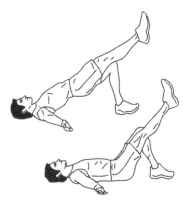

**10** one legged bridges

## 9    Aim to Misbehave

*"You all got on this boat for different reasons, but you all come to the same place. So now I'm asking more of you than I have before. Maybe all. Sure as I know anything I know this, they will try again. Maybe on another world, maybe on this very ground swept clean. A year from now, ten, they'll swing back to the belief that they can make people...better. And I do not hold to that. So no more running. I aim to misbehave. " Mal, Serenity*

**Focus: Strength &Tone, Upper Body**

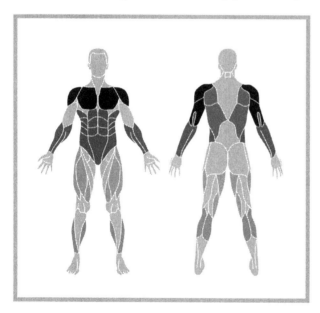

# I aim to misbehave

DAREBEE WORKOUT © darebee.com

**LEVEL I** 3 sets **LEVEL II** 4 sets **LEVEL III** 5 sets **REST** up to 2 minutes

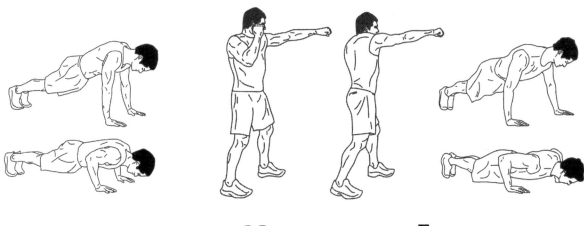

**5** push-ups          **20** punches          **5** wide grip push-ups

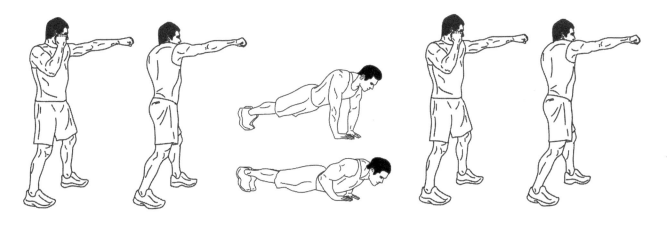

**20** punches          **5** close grip push-ups          **20** punches

# 10  Airborne

The floor is lava! Whatever you do, don't stay grounded. The Airborne Workout is a non-stop action and an at-home cardio routine that will work your entire body and challenge your aerobic capacity.

Take to the air to give wings to your performance afterwards in any kind of sporting activity. This is a workout that uses your bodyweight against you, maximizing the impact on your muscles for some pretty spectacular results.

**Focus: High Burn**

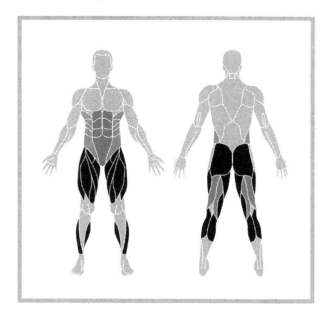

# AIRBORNE

DAREBEE WORKOUT © darebee.com

**LEVEL I** 3 sets  **LEVEL II** 5 sets  **LEVEL III** 7 sets  **REST** up to 2 minutes

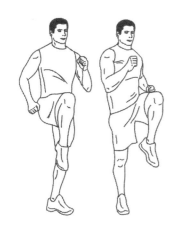

**20** high knees

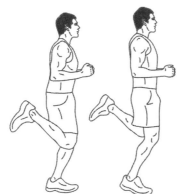

**10** butt kicks

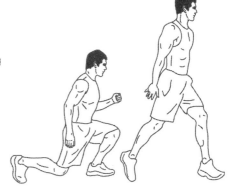

**10** jumping lunges

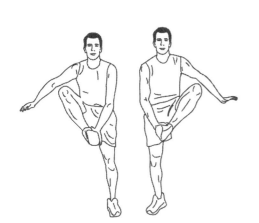

**20** toe tap hops

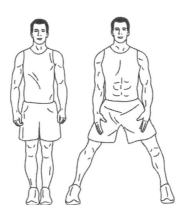

**10** half jacks

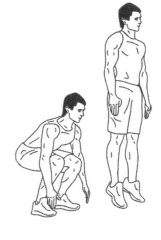

**10** jump squats

# 11    Amazon

Lower body strength, explosive moves, agility and grace are all part of the Amazon's armory of skills. This is a workout that pushes you from one peak to the other as successive exercises target muscle groups, making different demands on each one. Learn to combine different fitness attributes and seize control of your body.

**Focus: High Burn**

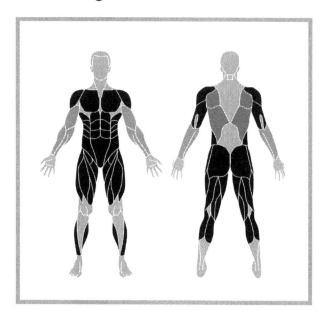

# AMAZON

DAREBEE WORKOUT © darebee.com

**LEVEL I** 3 sets  **LEVEL II** 5 sets  **LEVEL III** 7 sets  **REST** up to 2 minutes

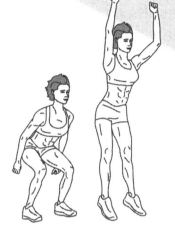

**10** jump squats

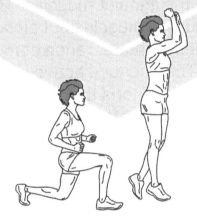

**10** jumping lunges

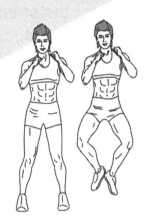

**10** hop heel clicks

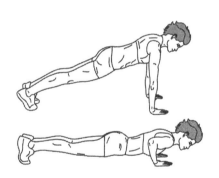

**10** push-ups

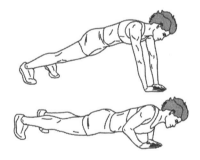

**2** close grip push-ups

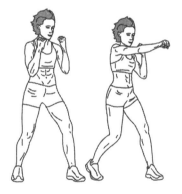

**20** punches

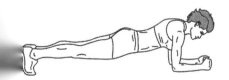

**20sec** elbow plank

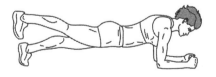

**20sec** raised leg plank

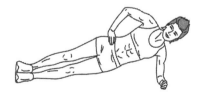

**20sec** side plank

## 12 Anchor'd

Active stretching demands you assume a position and then hold it using nothing but the strength of the agonist muscles. The results of active stretching are not just elongated muscles but also enhanced muscle growth, stronger tendons and a greater range of motion in the main muscle groups afterwards The Anchor'd active stretching workout takes you through some of the key positions that affect the body's main muscle groups. You will feel the difference afterwards.

**Focus: Stretching**

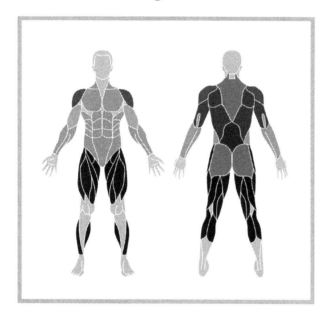

# ANCHOR'D

ACTIVE STRETCHING © darebee.com

**60 seconds each** - **30 seconds each leg**

**3 sets** | up to 2 minutes rest between sets

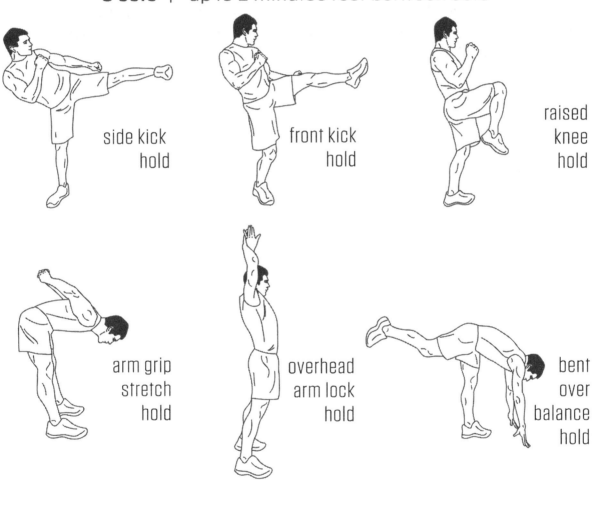

side kick
hold

front kick
hold

raised
knee
hold

arm grip
stretch
hold

overhead
arm lock
hold

bent
over
balance
hold

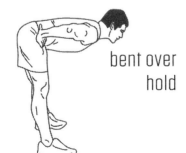

bent over
hold

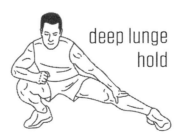

deep lunge
hold

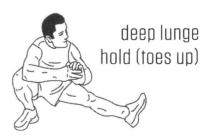

deep lunge
hold (toes up)

# 13 Armor Abs

A strong abdominal wall affects everything. The way you sit. How you walk. Your performance in every kind of sport. How quickly you get tired and how smoothly you move. This is a workout that presses all the right buttons, helping you tone up and build your abs, plus come summer you're going to be thankful you did it.

**Focus: Abs**

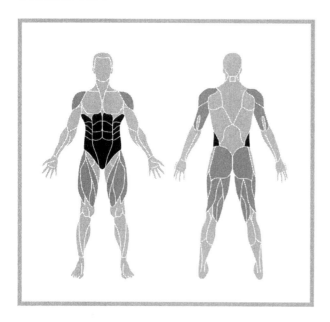

# armor abs

DAREBEE WORKOUT © darebee.com

**LEVEL I** 3 sets **LEVEL II** 5 sets **LEVEL III** 7 sets **REST** up to 2 minutes

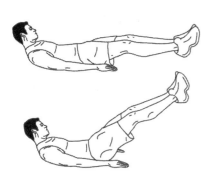

**10** leg raises

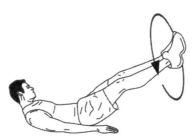

**10** raised leg circles

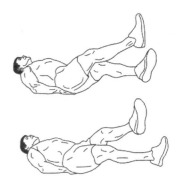

**10** scissors

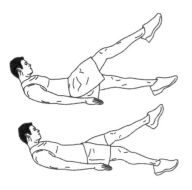

**20** flutter kicks

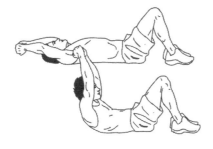

**5** long arm crunches

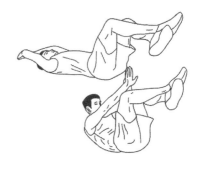

**5** knee crunches

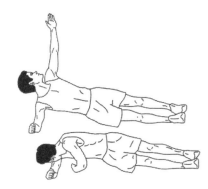

**10** side planks rotations

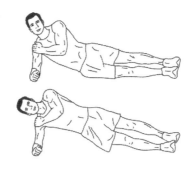

**10** side bridges

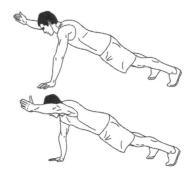

**10** plank arm raises

## 14 Arms of Steel

Whatever sport you may be doing, your arms are a critical component of it and the stronger they are, the better you get. Getting them strong however is not an easy job. This is where the Arms of Steel workout comes in. Not only does it tackle your arms from practically every angle but it also gives you no rest time, forcing your muscles to recover on the fly. Afterwards not only will you have arms of steel, you will also have the kind of arms that can power, manned, winged flight, almost.

**Focus: Strength & Tone, Upper Body**

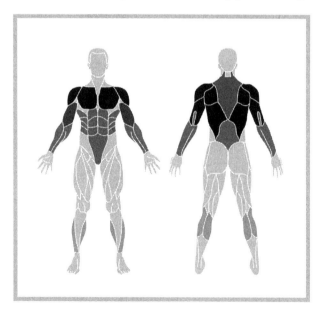

# Arms of Steel

DAREBEE WORKOUT © darebee.com

**LEVEL I** 3 sets  **LEVEL II** 4 sets  **LEVEL III** 5 sets  **REST** up to 2 minutes

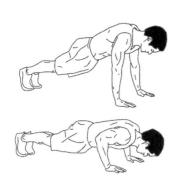

**10** push-ups

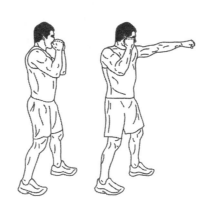

**20** punches

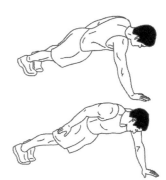

**10** thigh taps

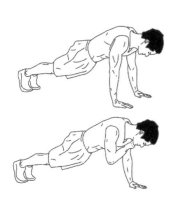

**10** shoulder taps

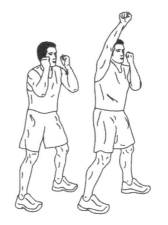

**20** overhead punches

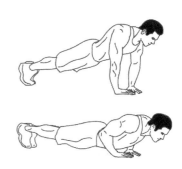

**10** tricep push-ups

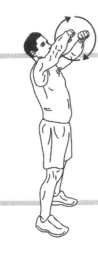

**2 minutes** rotating punches
aka speed bag punches
instead of complete rest after every set,
at any speed

# 15 Bacon

Also known as "The Belly Burner" workout this is designed to make you lean and mean. You will work up a sweat doing it. Your body will feel numb, your lungs will feel on fire and you will feel like you're being put through your paces. But ... you know it's worth it, and you're doing it for bacon. How cool is that?

**Focus: High Burn**

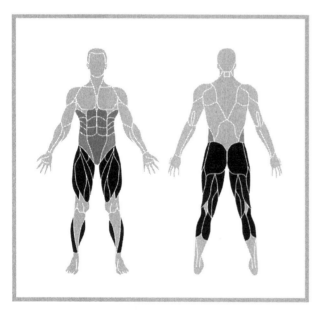

# YOU HAD ME AT
# bacon

DAREBEE WORKOUT © darebee.com

**LEVEL I** 3 sets **LEVEL II** 5 sets **LEVEL III** 7 sets **REST** up to 2 minutes

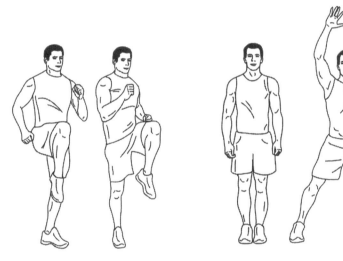

**40** high knees

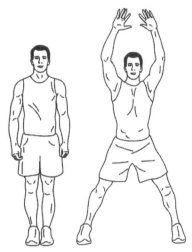

**10** jumping jacks

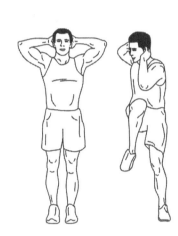

**10** knee-to-elbows

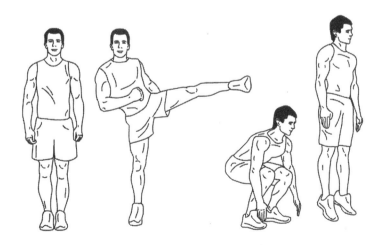

**40** side leg raises

**10** jump squats

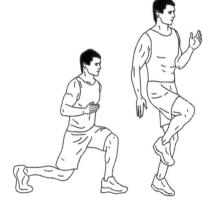

**10** lunge step-ups

## 16 Balance & Coordination

A good balance is the result of a strong core, stable tendons and powerful support muscle groups. Balance exercises help develop the muscle groups and tendons needed for developing muscular control, great physical prowess and the kind of body strength that marks true athletes.

**Focus: Strength / Balance**

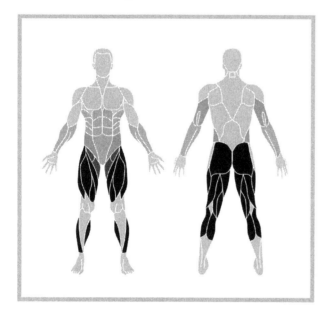

# BALANCE & COORDINATION

## DAREBEE WORKOUT © darebee.com

**LEVEL I** 3 sets  **LEVEL II** 5 sets  **LEVEL III** 7 sets  **REST** up to 2 minutes

Repeat the sequence going from one move to the next quickly
10 times in total (5 each side) = 1 set

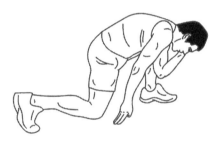

lunge

deep lunge elbow bent

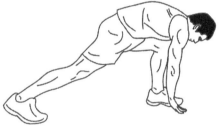

deep lunge

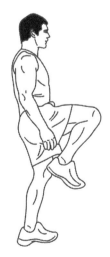

knee raise

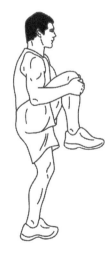

knee raise press

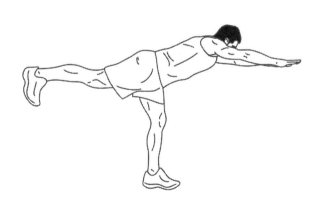

balance stand

## 17　Beast

You know the times when you need to contemplate life and need to get in touch with your spirit guide and discover your totem animal? This is just one of them. You get ready for action, look deep inside yourself and unleash your inner beast to help you get through the workout. In the process you discover a new you. Fresh capabilities are unlocked and muscles you probably haven't used before in quite the same way come into play and ... you transform.

**Focus: Strength & Tone**

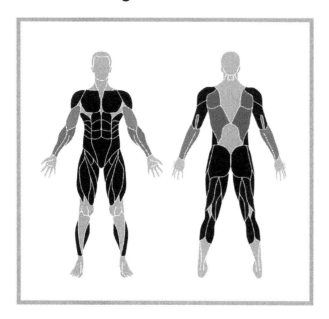

# the Beast

DAREBEE WORKOUT
© darebee.com
**LEVEL I** 3 sets
**LEVEL II** 5 sets
**LEVEL III** 7 sets
**REST** up to 2 minutes

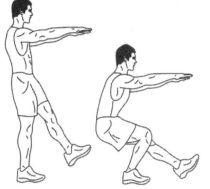

**20** pistol squats

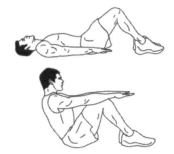

**20** sit-ups

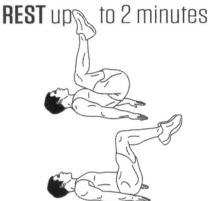

**20** reverse crunches

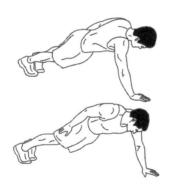

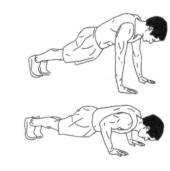

**10** push-ups

**20** thigh taps

**10** push-ups

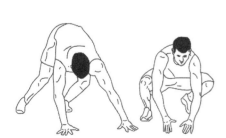

**10** side-to-side hops

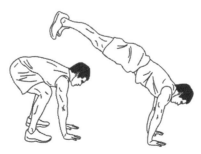

**10** back kicks

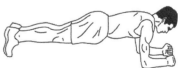

**60sec** plank

# 18 Bodyguard

Endurance is the capability of muscles to work long as well as hard. Like any athletic skill it can be developed. The Bodyguard workout helps you develop the ability to do sustained, high-energy work, long after everyone else around you has dropped to the ground with exhaustion.

**Focus: Strength & Tone**

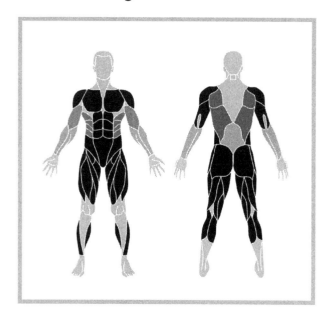

# BODYGUARD

DAREBEE WORKOUT © darebee.com

**LEVEL I** 3 sets  **LEVEL II** 5 sets  **LEVEL III** 7 sets  **REST** up to 2 minutes

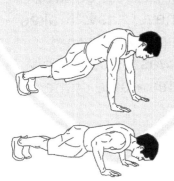

**20** push-ups

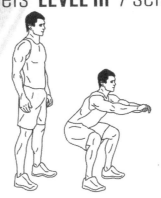

**40** squats

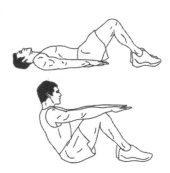

**40** sit-ups

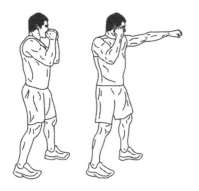

**40** punches

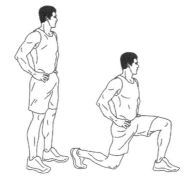

**40** lunges

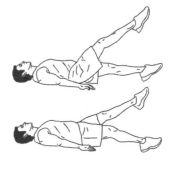

**40** flutter kicks

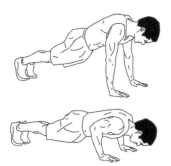

**20** push-ups

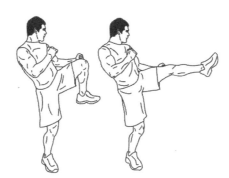

**40** front kicks

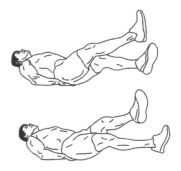

**40** scissors

# 19 Body Hack

We train because what we really want to do is hack our bodies. Control them. make them vehicles that do our bidding. That's never easy. It takes time, effort, hard work. The Body Hack workout is a step towards that direction: controlling the body you live in. If there ever was a rinse, apply, repeat formula that produced the desirable outcome, this would come pretty close to being it.

**Focus: Strength & Tone**

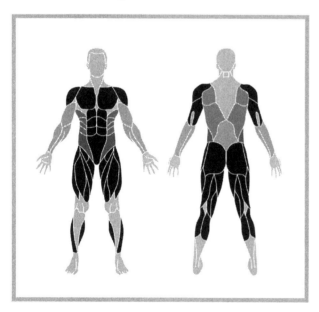

# BODY HACK

## DAREBEE WORKOUT © darebee.com

**LEVEL I** 3 sets  **LEVEL II** 5 sets  **LEVEL III** 7 sets  **REST** up to 2 minutes

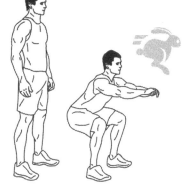

**10** fast squats

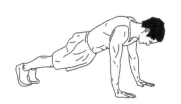

**10-count** plank

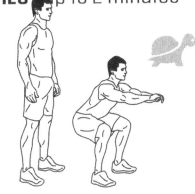

**10** slow squats

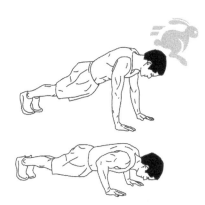

**5** fast push-ups

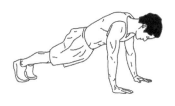

**10-count** plank

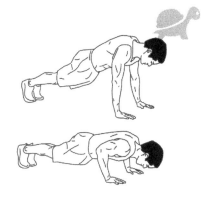

**5** slow push-ups

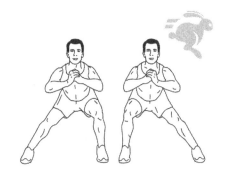

**10** fast side-to-side lunges

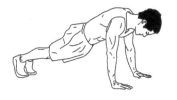

**10-count** plank

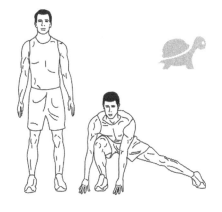

**10** slow side lunges

# 20 Borderline

The only time a borderline workout can be improved is when it involves two lines, instead of just one. Now I know you think things cannot get any better but trust me, the moment you have two lines on the floor to deal with, the intensity of the workout changes completely.

**Focus: High Burn**

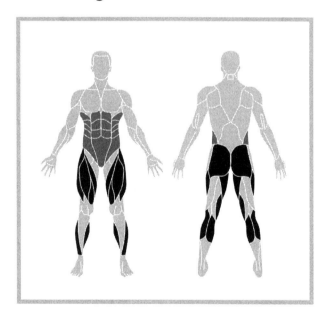

# BORDERLINE 2.0

DAREBEE WORKOUT © darebee.com

**LEVEL I** 3 sets **LEVEL II** 5 sets **LEVEL III** 7 sets **REST** up to 2 minutes

draw two lines shoulder length apart

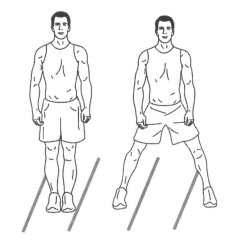

**20** half jacks
jump-inside the lines

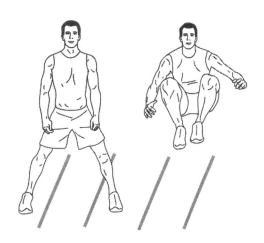

**10** high jumps
with heel click in the air

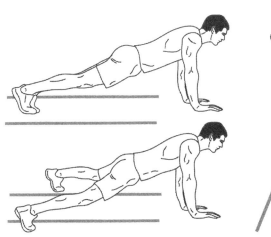

**10** plank half jacks
jump inside the lines

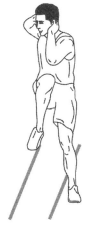

**10** knee to elbow
across the lines

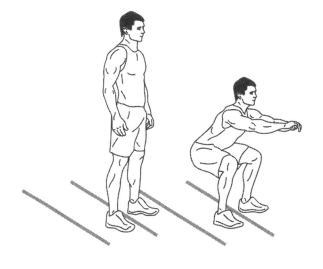

**20** over the line step
side-to-side squats

# 21 Boulder

Strength is not just about muscle size. It depends on muscle density, the type of muscle fiber you have. The composition of each bundle of muscle and its ability to perform under physical stress. The Boulder workout definitely creates some physical stress to challenge the muscles so you get to feel like a rock.

**Focus: Strength & Tone**

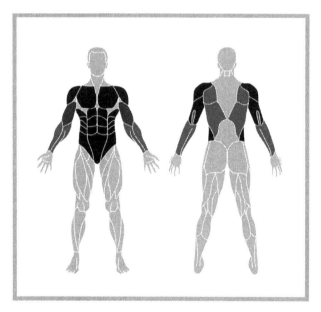

# THE BOULDER

DAREBEE WORKOUT © darebee.com

**LEVEL I** 3 sets  **LEVEL II** 5 sets  **LEVEL III** 7 sets  **REST** up to 2 minutes

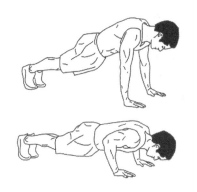

**10** push-ups

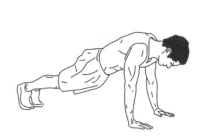

**10-count** plank

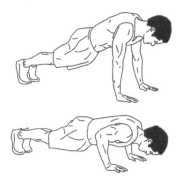

**10** push-ups

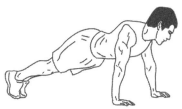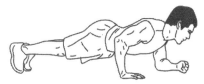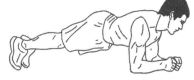

**10** up and down planks

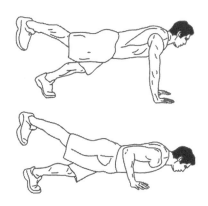

**10** raised leg push-ups

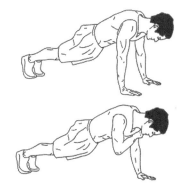

**10** shoulder taps

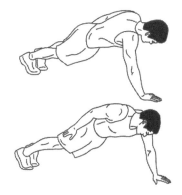

**10** thigh taps

# 22 Boxer

Boxers have blazingly-fast hands, incredible stamina, focus, strength, perseverance, the ability to compartmentalize pain and great spatial awareness. All of which can now be yours provided you use this workout to remake your body and transform your spirit. Plus, when you next hear the Rocky soundtrack you'll be able to deservedly throw your arms up towards the sky and jog on the spot (com'on, you know you want to).

**Focus: Strength & Tone**

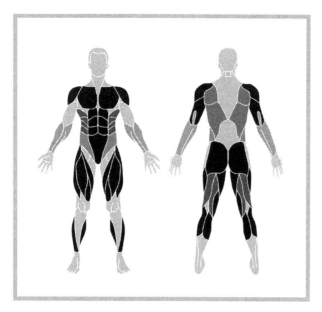

# BOXER

**5 SETS** DAREBEE WORKOUT © darebee.com
up to 2 minutes rest between rounds

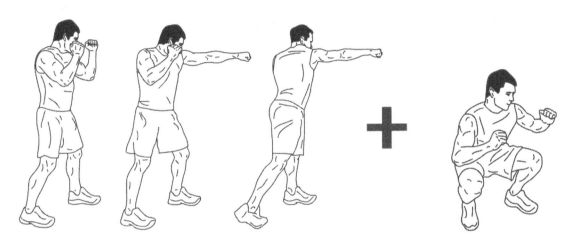

**5 minute** shadow boxing       **every 30 seconds** double squat

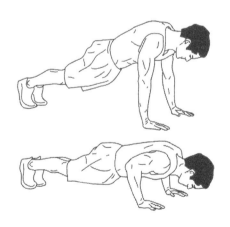

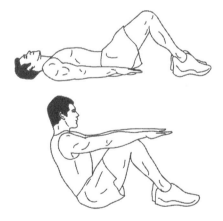

**push-ups**
**level I** 5 reps
**level II** 10 reps
**level III** 15 reps

**sit-ups**
**level I** 10 reps
**level II** 20 reps
**level III** 30 reps

# 23    Boxer HIIT

Boxers have phenomenal limb speed, arm strength and stamina. They can generate tremendous forces on the areas they strike and are easily amongst the most fearsome unarmed fighters anyone can hope to face. The Boxer HIIT workout combines some of the favourite moves of boxing with a high intensity interval training plan that will push your body to its limits.

**Focus: High Burn, HIIT**

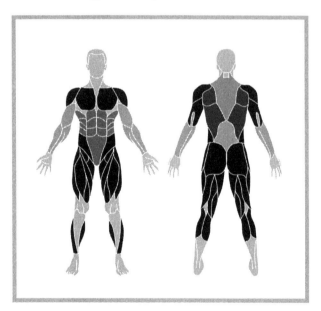

# BOXER

DAREBEE `HIIT` WORKOUT © **darebee.com**

**Level I**   5 rounds   **Level II**   10 rounds   **Level III**   15 rounds
1 minute rest between rounds

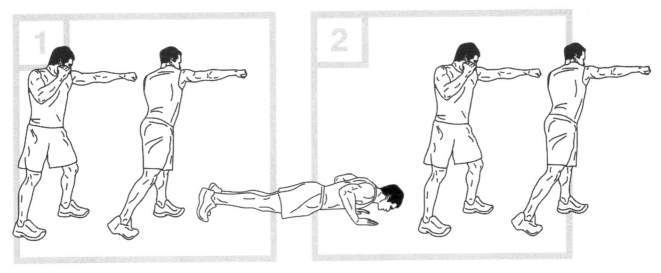

**20sec** jab + cross          **20sec** push-up + jab + cross

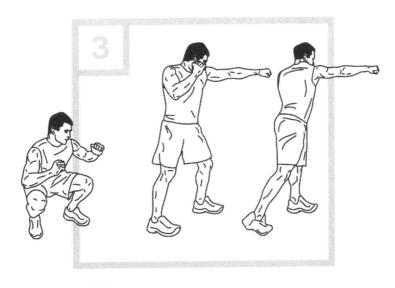

**20sec** squat + jab + cross

# 24 Boy, that escalated

There are days when all you want to do is empty your mind and then 'empty' your body into an activity that simply works you physically until you're done. Well, look no further than this workout for that. It may not appear very challenging at first glance but you will find that it presses all the right buttons.

**Focus: High Burn**

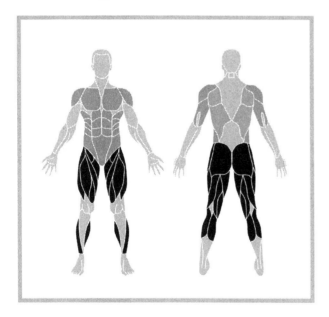

# BOY, THAT ESCALATED QUICKLY

DAREBEE WORKOUT
© darebee.com

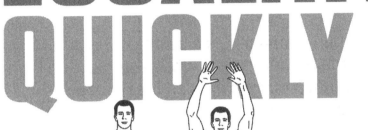

**10** jumping jacks
**10** high knees
**4** side-to-side jumps

**20** jumping jacks
**20** high knees
**4** side-to-side jumps

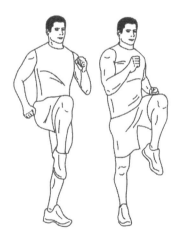

**40** jumping jacks
**40** high knees
**4** side-to-side jumps

done

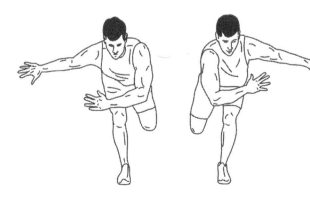

**LEVEL I**   3 sets
**LEVEL II**  5 sets
**LEVEL III** 7 sets
**REST** up to 2 minutes

## 25  Cardio & Core

At the core of every great athletic performance lies a strong core (pun unintended) and great cardiovascular conditioning. While aerobic performance determines just how much oxygen in each breath you take is really absorbed by the lungs and transferred into the bloodstream to be taken to the organs that need it, cardiovascular fitness is the ability of the heart and lungs to get all the blood circulating quickly enough through the body to supply oxygen to the organs and tissues that need it most. The Cardio & Core workout puts your body through its paces testing your core and challenging your cardiovascular fitness. All you have to do now is supply the great athletic performance.

**Focus: High Burn**

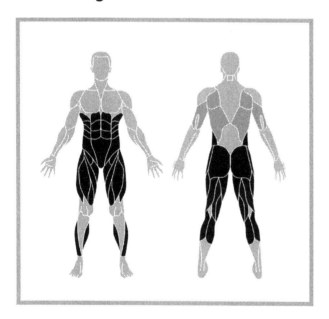

# Cardio & Core

DAREBEE WORKOUT © darebee.com

**LEVEL I** 3 sets  **LEVEL II** 5 sets  **LEVEL III** 7 sets  **REST** up to 2 minutes

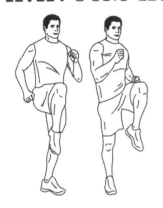

**60** high knees

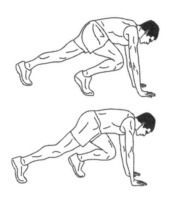

**10** climbers

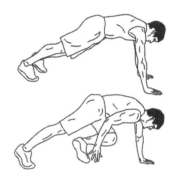

**10** climber taps

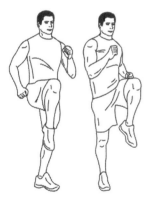

**60** high knees

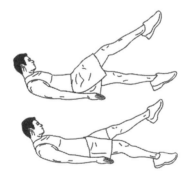

**10** flutter kicks

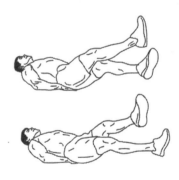

**10** scissors

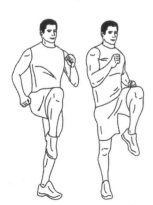

**60** high knees

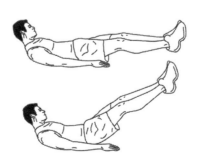

**10** leg raises

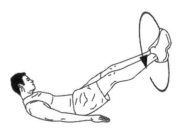

**10** raised leg circles

# 26 Chisel

Getting that chiseled physique requires patience, perseverance and the ability to put in the time one day after another. Chisel, of course, is the workout that'll help you do all this. A combination of aerobic and strength exercises it works all the major muscle groups so that your body keeps on changing the way you want it to.

**Focus: High Burn**

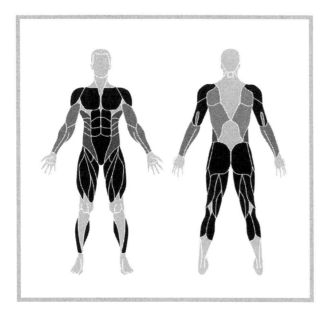

# CHISEL

DAREBEE WORKOUT © darebee.com

**LEVEL I** 3 sets **LEVEL II** 5 sets **LEVEL III** 7 sets **REST** up to 2 minutes

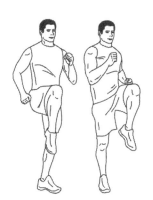

**20** high knees

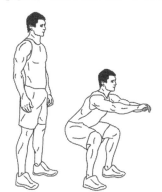

**10** squats

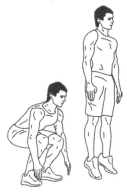

**10** jump squats

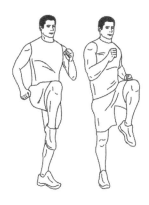

**20** high knees

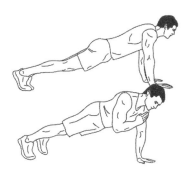

**10** shoulder taps

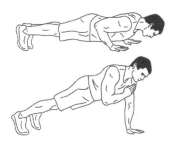

**10** shoulder tap push-ups

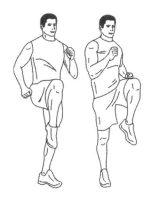

**20** high knees

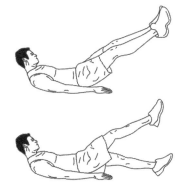

**10** flutter kicks

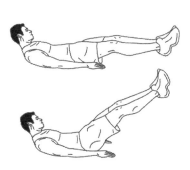

**10** leg raises

# 27 Close Contact

When things get up close and personal your body is the only thing that keeps you alive. The Close Contact workout transforms you into a living, breathing fighting machine. The moves are biomechanically optimized. The results are a workout that pushes strength, speed, power, agility, coordination and control. Not quite the perfect workout but darned close.

**Focus: High Burn**

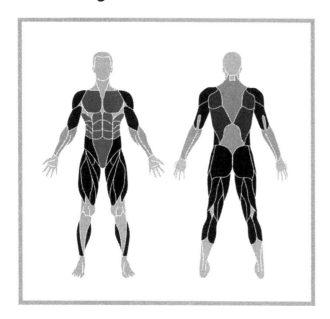

# CLOSE CONTACT

DAREBEE WORKOUT © darebee.com

**LEVEL I** 3 sets **LEVEL II** 5 sets **LEVEL III** 7 sets **REST** up to 2 minutes

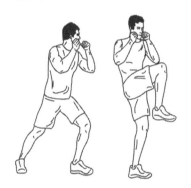 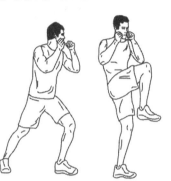

**20** knee strikes          **20combo** knee strike + elbow strike

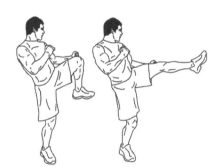 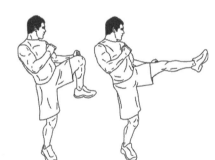

**20** front kicks          **20combos** front kick + backfist

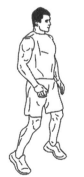 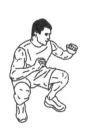 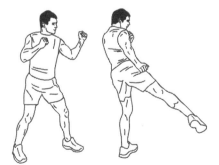 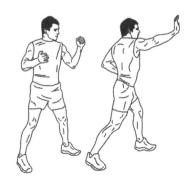

**20combos** bounce + squat + back leg low turning kick + palm strike

# 28  Code of Abs

The code, the source code. Strong abs are not just the engine that powers your every move nor are they just the armour that protects some of your vital organs. They're also the scaffolding that supports your spine. In short they're really important. That's why you need them. Plus they make you look cool when you take your shirt off.

**Focus: Abs**

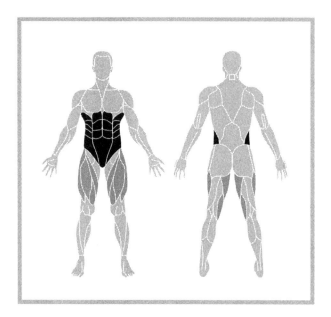

# code of abs

DAREBEE WORKOUT © darebee.com

**LEVEL I** 3 sets **LEVEL II** 4 sets **LEVEL III** 5 sets **REST** up to 2 minutes

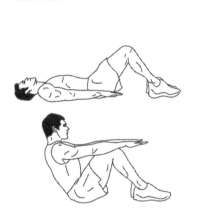

**10** sit-ups

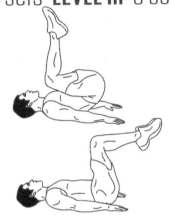

**10** reverse crunches

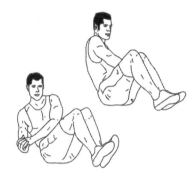

**10** sitting twists

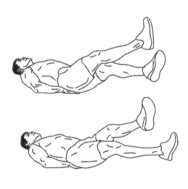

**8** scissors

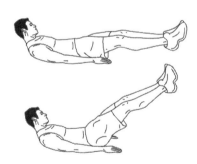

**8** leg raises

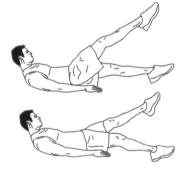

**20** flutter kicks

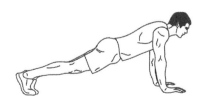

**30sec** plank

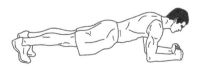

**30sec** elbow plank

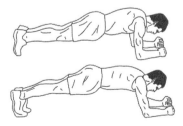

**8** body saw

## 29    Codex

Stay glued to the ground and see just how much you can challenge your body. This is a set of exercises that takes a traditional routine and gives it an extra spin with a real challenge. Because of that it forces your muscles to work in unfamiliar ways that make it totally challenging.

**Focus: High Burn**

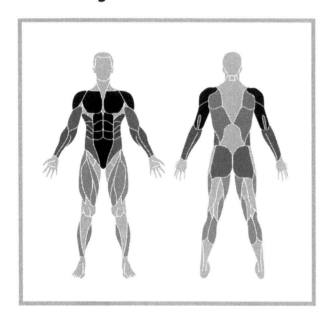

# CODEX

DAREBEE WORKOUT © darebee.com

**LEVEL I** 3 sets **LEVEL II** 5 sets **LEVEL III** 7 sets **REST** up to 2 minutes
hands never off the ground

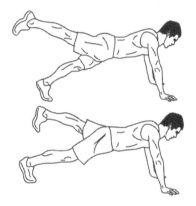

**10** plank leg raises

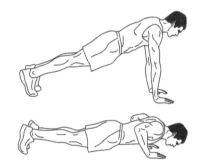

**10** push-ups

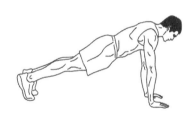

**30sec** plank

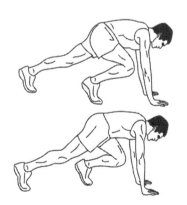

**10** climbers

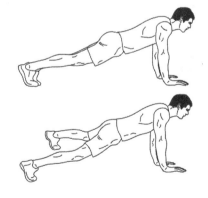

**10** plank jacks

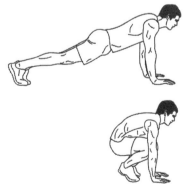

**10** plank jump-ins

## 30 Coffee Break

A coffee break is always great, especially if your day starts with one, which then doesn't quite make it a break but there is certainly coffee involved. Add some movement, throw in a little need for balance and you've got yourself the kind of workout Kung Fu legends are made of. Fill your cup almost to the brim and you're beginning to get into the Jedi zone. The Coffee Break workout may not look that challenging at first glance but try it out with a cup that's filled almost to the brim and you will find it takes incredible and muscle control to prevent it from spilling. Exactly the kind of balance and muscle control that allow you to move with the sureness of a panther and the speed of a snake. Now go get that cup of coffee.

**Focus: High Burn**

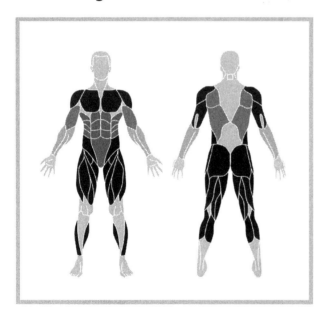

# Coffee BREAK

DAREBEE WORKOUT © darebee.com

**3 sets** | up to 2 minutes rest between sets

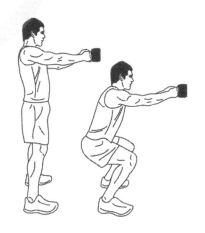

**10** squats

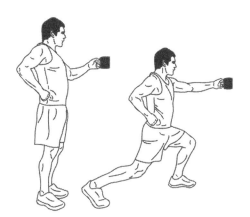

**10** lunges

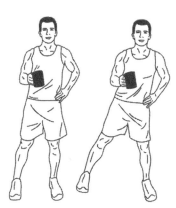

**10** side leg swings

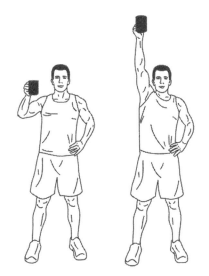

**20** mug raises

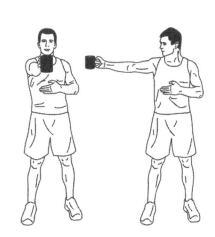

**20** arm rotations

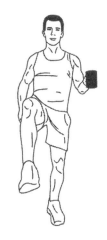

**20-count** hold

# 31 Combat Strength

Turn your body into a pillar of strength, capable of almost anything with the Combat Strength workout. As the name suggests the aim is to challenge major muscle groups building up the strength and speed you'd need in a hypothetical combat scenario where all you have is your body and the razor-sharp mind that guides it.

**Focus: Strength & Tone**

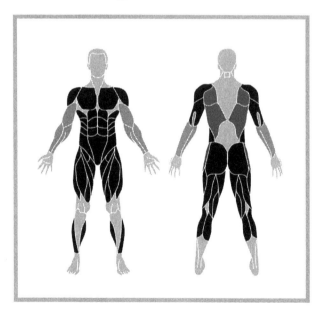

# Combat Strength

DAREBEE WORKOUT © darebee.com

**LEVEL I** 3 sets   **LEVEL II** 5 sets   **LEVEL III** 7 sets   **REST** up to 2 minutes

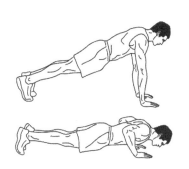

**10** push-ups

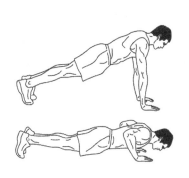

**10combos** push-up + jab + cross

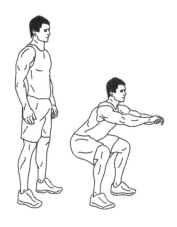

**10** squats

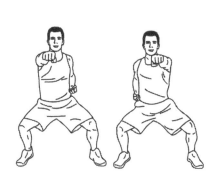

**40** squat hold punches

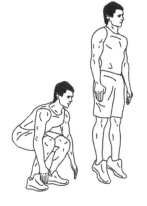

**10** jump squats

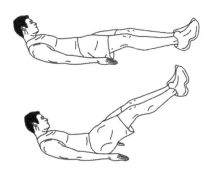

**20** leg raises

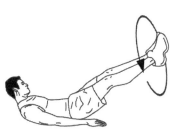

**20** raised leg circles

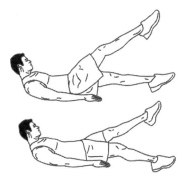

**20** flutter kicks

# 32   Contender

One of the hardest things you can do is get into a ring and go a few rounds. Beyond the fact that there is the inevitable exchange of blows you are pushing your entire body to the limit with no room to ease off, no matter how much your muscles ache or your lungs burn. As a physical test the Contender takes you through one exercise after another, slowly loading each muscle group and then asking you to exercise even as fatigue tags at you. Well, there is no exchange of blows taking place, so dig deep and feel the burn.

**Focus: Strength & Tone**

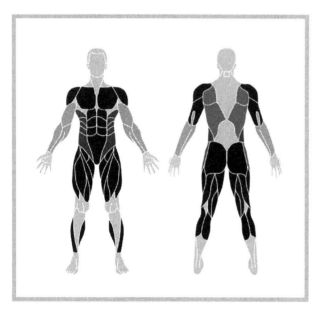

# CONTENDER

DAREBEE WORKOUT © darebee.com

**LEVEL I** 3 sets  **LEVEL II** 5 sets  **LEVEL III** 7 sets  **REST** up to 2 minutes

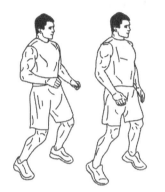

**30** bounces

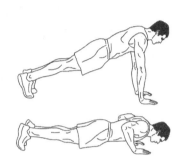

**5** push-ups

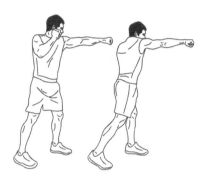

**30** punches

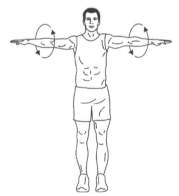

**30** arm rotations

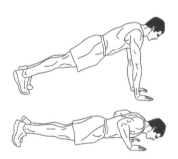

**5** push-ups

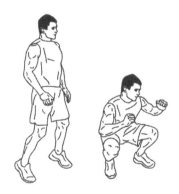

**30** squats

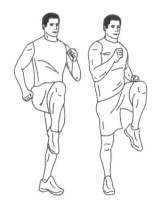

**30** high knees

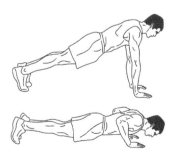

**5** push-ups

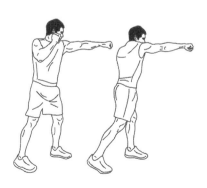

**30** punches

## 33   Core Connect

A strong core is not easy to come by. The muscles associated with it (transversus abdominis) help develop better functional movements and prevent injury. The core is active in both static and dynamic movements as it brings the skeletal structure into play and allows it to align itself so that it can better absorb and direct specific forces. The Core Connect workout helps strengthen your core and change the way you do, everything.

**Focus: Abs & Core**

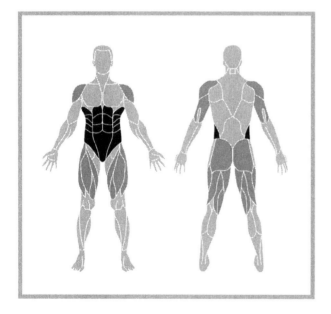

# core connect

DAREBEE WORKOUT © darebee.com

**LEVEL I** 3 sets **LEVEL II** 5 sets **LEVEL III** 7 sets **REST** up to 2 minutes
**10 reps each exercise**

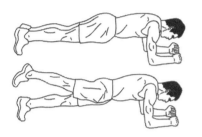

plank leg raises

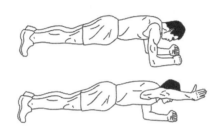

plank arm raises

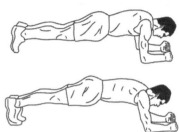

body saw

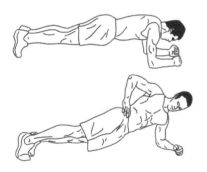

plank rotations

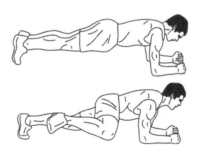

spiderman planks

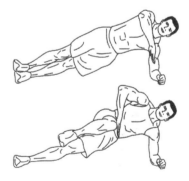

side plank knee taps

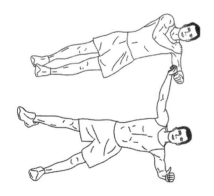

side star plank

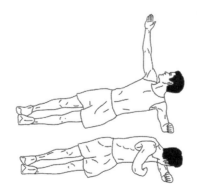

side plank rotations

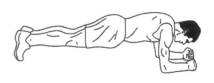

**to failure** elbow plank

## 34  Crucible

For those who have played Destiny once or twice, the Crucible is a place where Guardians go to test their skills and cement their reputations. This Crucible is a little different, no skills or armor will be gained by doing the workout but your reputation might well be cemented.

**Focus: Strength & Tone**

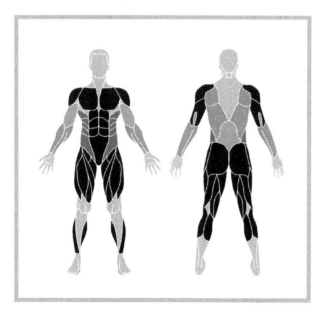

# CRUCIBLE

**DAREBEE WORKOUT © darebee.com**

**LEVEL I** 5 push-ups **LEVEL II** 10 push-ups **LEVEL III** 15 push-ups
**LEVEL I** 3 sets **LEVEL II** 5 sets **LEVEL III** 7 sets **REST** up to 2 minutes

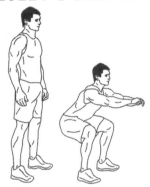

**20** squats

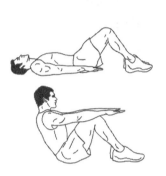

**10** sit-ups

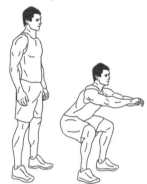

**20** squats

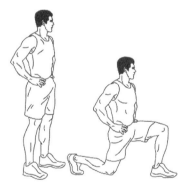

**20** lunges

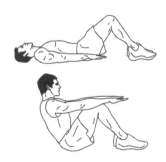

**10** sit-ups

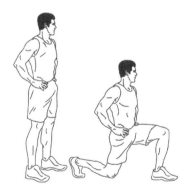

**20** lunges

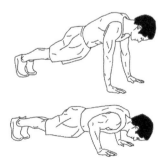

**X** push-ups

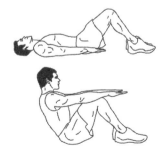

**10** sit-ups

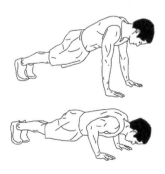

**X** push-ups

## 35 Daily Burn

On those great, exceptional days when you leap out of bed with a fire in your belly and a song in your heart you know that through physical training you "forge your body to the fire of your will". Every other day you just need to purse your lips and get on with it in a workout that'll work for you. Well this is the one for those unexceptional days.

**Focus: High Burn**

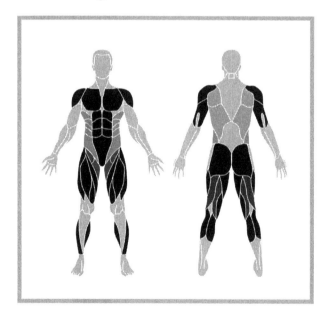

# Daily Burn

DAREBEE WORKOUT © darebee.com

**3 sets** | up to 2 minutes rest between sets

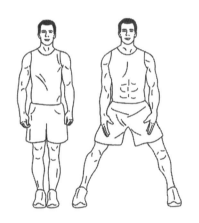

**10** half jacks

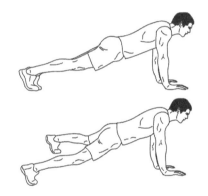

**6** plank jacks

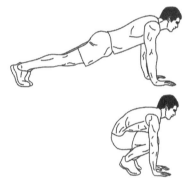

**6** plank jump-ins

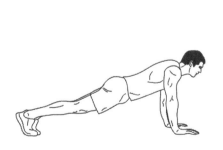

**10-count** plank

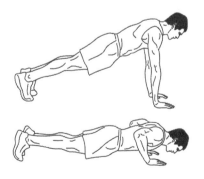

**6** push-ups

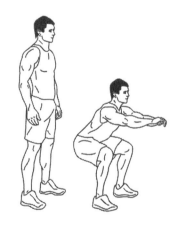

**10** squats

## 36    Daily Workout

This is the perfect workout for those days when you're not sure what to do and know you really need to do something to workout. Use it as a filler, a routine, the go-to work out when you have nothing else to fire you up. At ten reps per exercise there really is no excuse not to do them.

**Focus: High Burn**

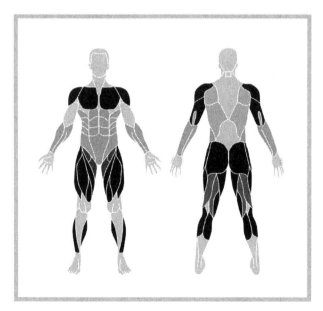

# DAILY WORKOUT

BY DAREBEE © darebee.com

**3 sets** | up to 2 minutes rest between sets

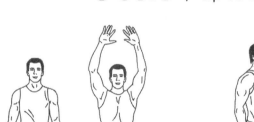

**10** jumping jacks

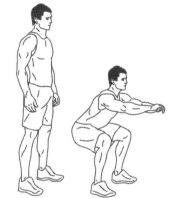

**5** squats

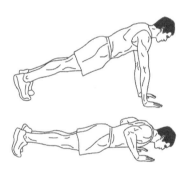

**5** push-ups

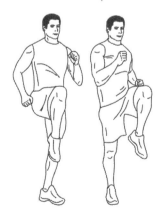

**10** high knees

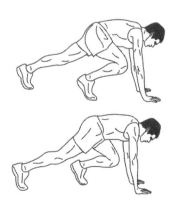

**10** climbers

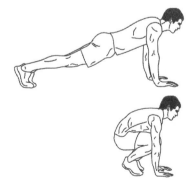

**5** plank jump-ins

## 37 Dash

Building up speed relies on forcing muscles to undergo a few adaptive changes. There are two parts to becoming lightning-fast, the first part requires developing the muscle structure itself, increasing the number of neurons and developing fast-twitch action fiber. The second part requires strengthening of all the supporting muscle groups and tendons that help major muscle groups perform. The DASH workout is designed to help you develop both. Each exercise is performed at full speed.

**Focus: High Burn**

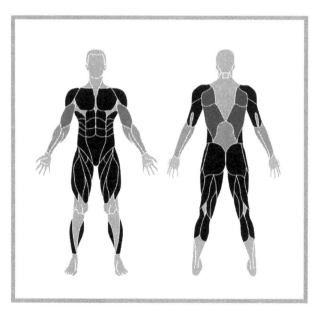

# DASH

DAREBEE WORKOUT © darebee.com

**LEVEL I** 3 sets **LEVEL II** 5 sets **LEVEL III** 7 sets **REST** up to 2 minutes

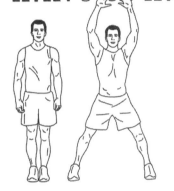

**20** jumping jacks

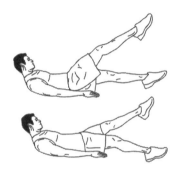

**10** flutter kicks

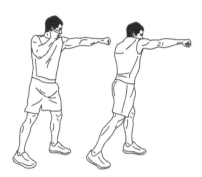

**40** punches

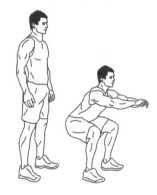

**20** squats

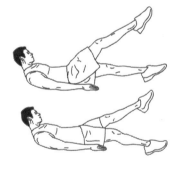

**10** flutter kicks

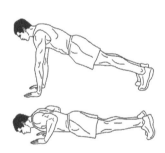

**10** push-ups

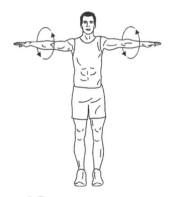

**40** raised arm circles

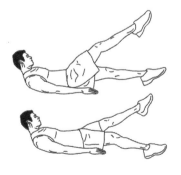

**10** flutter kicks

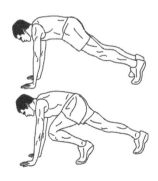

**10** climbers

## 38 DNA: rewrite

What if you could transform yourself into the kind of physically capable person you want to be? How would you rewrite your DNA? This is a workout that helps you explore the possibilities lying at the boundaries of your capabilities.

**Focus: High Burn**

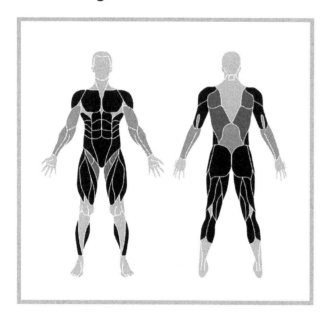

# DNA:REWRITE

DAREBEE WORKOUT © darebee.com

**LEVEL I** 3 sets **LEVEL II** 5 sets **LEVEL III** 7 sets **REST** up to 2 minutes

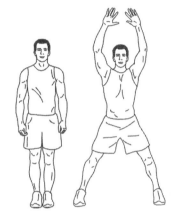

**10** jumping jacks

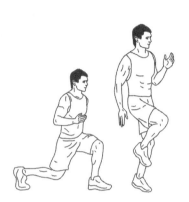

**10** lunge step-ups

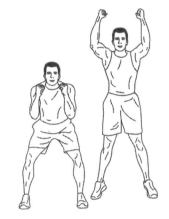

**10** jumps

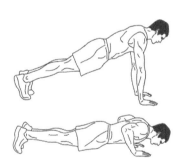

**10** push-ups

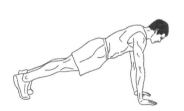

**10-count** plank

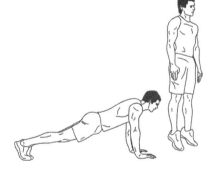

**10** basic burpees w/ jump

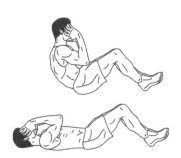

**10** sit-ups

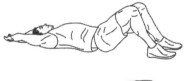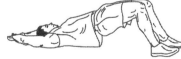

**10** bridges

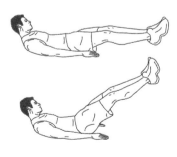

**10** leg raises

# 39  Double Up

You have two arms which means you will be experiencing twice the joy as the Double Up workout uses the rapid motion of the arms to also challenge the core and abs and even your glutes and quads and hamstrings. The amazing thing about the connected body is that the upper body powers the lower body so strong arms help you run faster, longer and the lower body powers the upper one so that strong legs help you punch harder.

**Focus: High Burn**

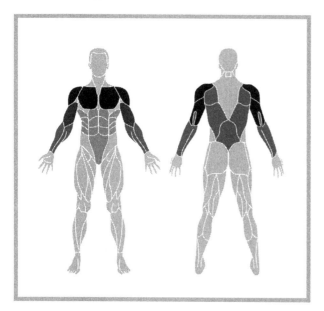

# DOUBLE UP

DAREBEE WORKOUT © darebee.com

**LEVEL I** 3 sets **LEVEL II** 5 sets **LEVEL III** 7 sets **REST** up to 2 minutes

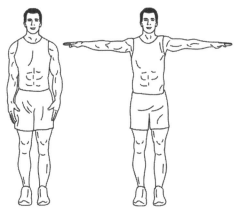

**20** side arm raises

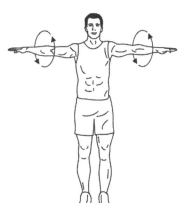

**20** raised arm circles

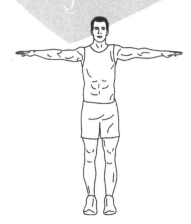

**20-count** arm hold

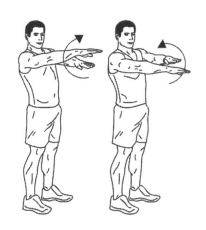

**20** fast scissors

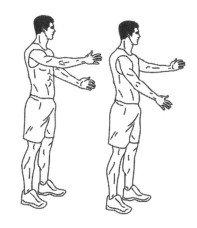

**20** scissor chops

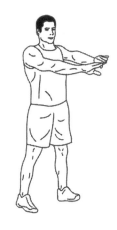

**20-count** arm hold

## 40   Dynamic Pyramid

Pyramid workouts are great because they work overlapping but separate systems in your body. Your cardiovascular, anaerobic and aerobic systems are worked here which means that you also get to build up some serious endurance.

**Focus: High Burn**

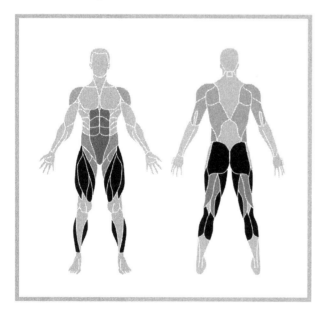

# dynamic
# pyramid

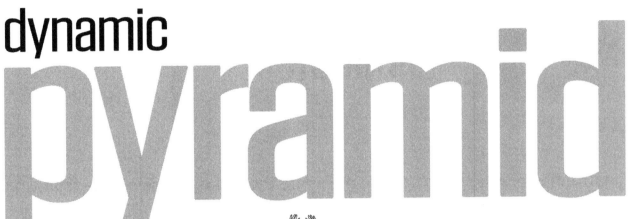

DAREBEE WORKOUT
ⓒ darebee.com
**LEVEL I** 3 sets
**LEVEL II** 5 sets
**LEVEL III** 7 sets
**REST** up to 2 minutes

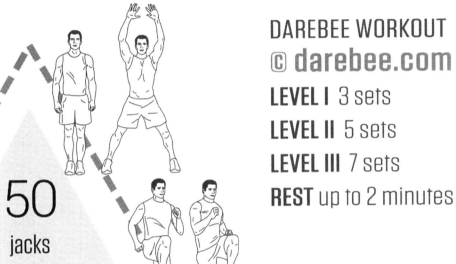

50 jacks

40 high knees 40

30 climbers 30

20 squats 20

0 plank jump-ins 10

## 41 Eliminator

Instructions: After each set you eliminate the last exercise off the following set, the goal is to do enough sets to get to doing nothing. Yay!

**Focus: High Burn**

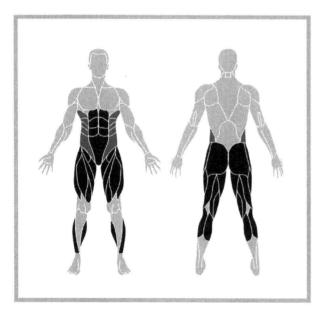

# X ELIMINATOR

DAREBEE WORKOUT © darebee.com

**5 sets** – after every set take the last exercise off the following set

**rest between sets** up to 45 seconds

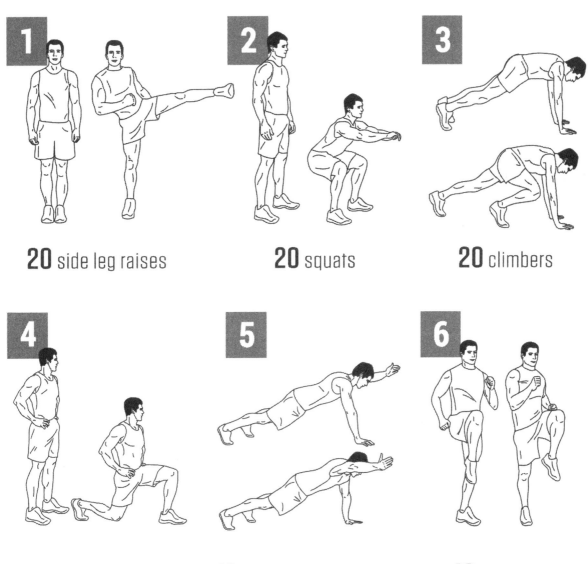

**20** side leg raises

**20** squats

**20** climbers

**20** lunges

**10** plank arm raises

**40** high knees

## 42 Epic

This is a simple, alternating, high-burn workout that will leave you out of breath and feeling like you're worthy of the title of "Epic". Do each rep to the max and just enjoy the journey.

**Focus: Strength & Tone**

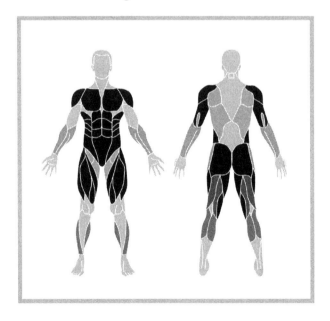

# EPIC QUEST

DAREBEE WORKOUT © darebee.com

**LEVEL I** 3 sets **LEVEL II** 5 sets **LEVEL III** 7 sets **REST** up to 2 minutes

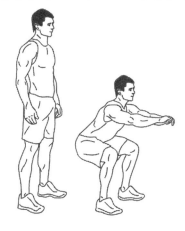

**20** squats
**20** knee-to-elbow crunches

**10** push-ups
**10** knee-to-elbow crunches

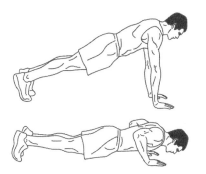

**20** squats
**20** knee-to-elbow crunches

**10** push-ups
**10** knee-to-elbow crunches

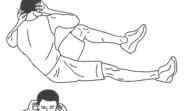

**20** squats
**20** knee-to-elbow crunches

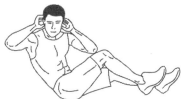

**10** push-ups
**10** knee-to-elbow crunches

## 43   Express

This is the workout for when you want something fast, are pressed for time but don't want to skimp on quality. Up the intensity just a little on each rep and you can both have your cake and eat it.

**Focus: Strength & Tone**

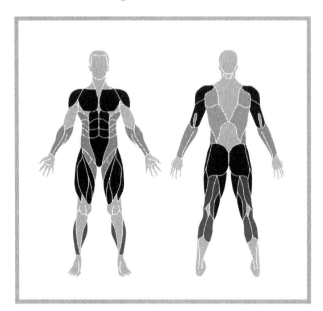

# EXPRESS
## WORKOUT
BY DAREBEE © darebee.com

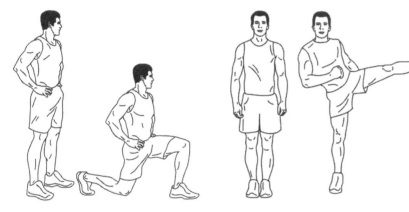

**20** lunges

**20** side leg raises

**20** squats

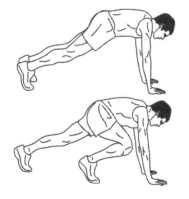

**20** slow climber

**20** push-ups

**20sec** elbow plank

## 44 Extractor

There are some days when all you want to do is go through a workout where you do not have to think much, or concentrate hard. You take yourself out of the picture and let your body do its thing. The Extractor workout is just the thing that will do that for you.

**Focus: High Burn**

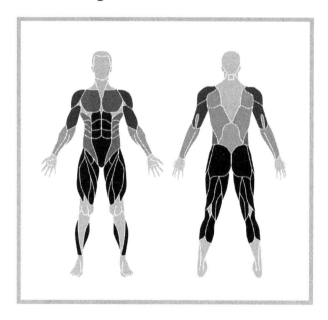

# EXTRACTOR

DAREBEE WORKOUT © darebee.com

**LEVEL I** 3 sets  **LEVEL II** 5 sets  **LEVEL III** 7 sets  **REST** up to 2 minutes

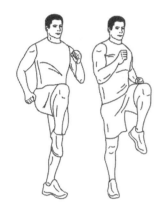

**20** high knees

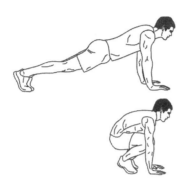

**5** plank jump-ins

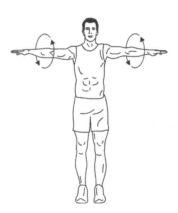

**20** raised arm circles

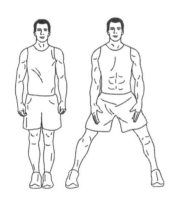

**20** half jacks

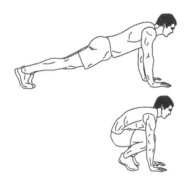

**5** plank jump-ins

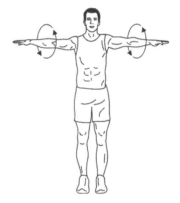

**20** raised arm circles

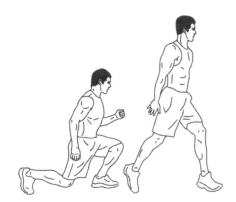

**20** jumping lunges

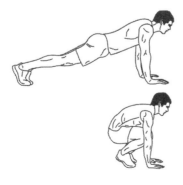

**5** plank jump-ins

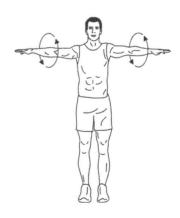

**20** raised arm circles

## 45 Far Point

Passive stretching is an ideal form of stretching to perform with a partner. It requires the body to remain completely passive while an outside force is exerted upon it (by a partner). When used without a partner bodyweight and the force of gravity are allowed to do their thing. Passive stretching is also called relaxed stretching, for that reason. To make it work for you, extend to a position that is at the very edge of your comfort zone and hold it, allowing gravity and your bodyweight to do the rest. There is no 'bounce' of any kind with passive stretching, nor is there any push/pull motion. Find out more about Stretching for Strength and Flexibility.

**Focus: Stretching**

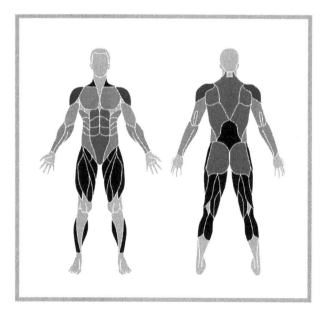

# FAR POINT

PASSIVE STRETCHING © darebee.com

**60 seconds each** - **30 seconds each side / leg**

**3 sets** | up to 2 minutes rest between sets

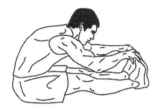

hamstring stretch

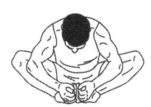

groin stretch

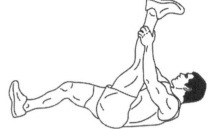

leg to chest stretch

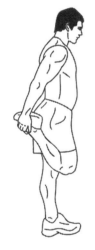

quad stretch

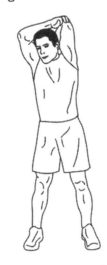

elbow stretch

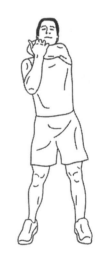

cross neck elbow stretch

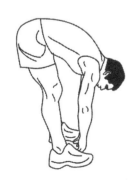

gravity toe touches

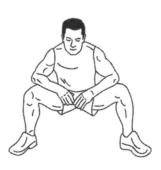

sumo squat hold

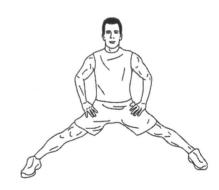

side splits

# 46  Five Minute Plank

Training the abdominal muscle group is no easy task. The muscles do not all respond to training at the same rate and there is a core group of abdominal s, running beneath the external ones with muscle fibres pointing the opposite way. This makes for a core picture which no single exercise can adequately address which helps explain why strong abs are hard to attain, which makes them an aim to strive for.

The five minute plank is a paradox of sorts. It uses relative inactivity to challenge the abdominal muscles and strengthen them. In five minutes you get to exercise as many parts as possible of the muscle wall. The result: strong abs, a strong core, more power, better coordination plus you get to look good on the beach.

**Focus: Abs**

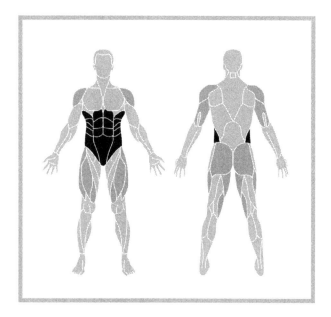

# FIVE MINUTE PLANK

DAREBEE WORKOUT © darebee.com

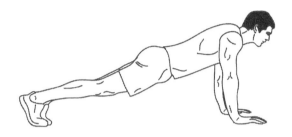

**60sec** full plank

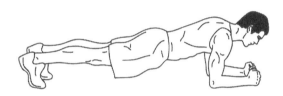

**30sec** elbow plank

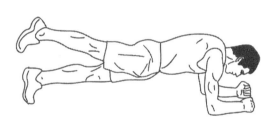

**60sec** raised leg plank
30 seconds - each leg

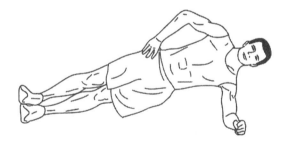

**60sec** side plank
30 seconds - each side

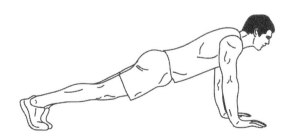

**30sec** full plank

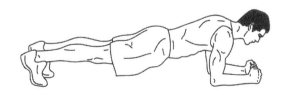

**60sec** elbow plank

## 47 Flash Point

Everyone wants to get their body to the point where the muscles just 'catch on fire' and they become a smooth blur of movement. The Flashpoint workout helps you do just this. Based on martial arts combinations it activates all the important muscle groups plus supporting muscle structures for a truly holistic workout.

**Focus: High Burn**

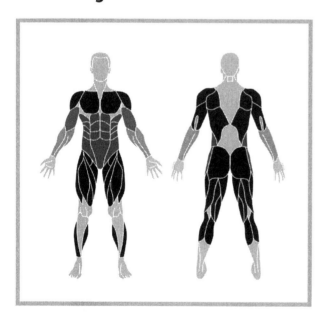

# Flash Point

DAREBEE WORKOUT © darebee.com

**LEVEL I** 3 sets **LEVEL II** 5 sets **LEVEL III** 7 sets **REST** up to 2 minutes

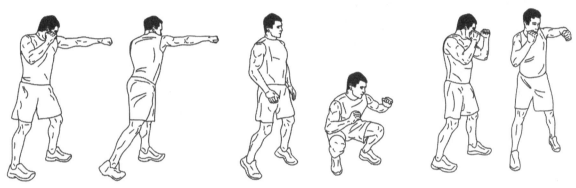

**40 combos** jab + cross + squat + hook

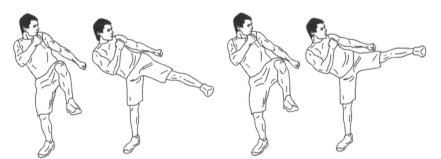

**40** double side kicks / low and high

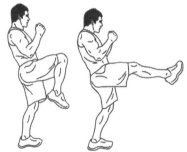

**40** front kicks

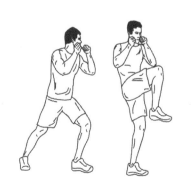

**40 combos** knee strike + elbow strike

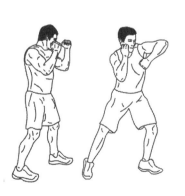

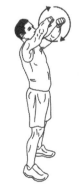

**40** speed bag punches

## 48 Fremen

When you're destined to be amongst the best fighters in the Universe from birth, physical fitness is a way of life. The Spice will make that life long but just how awesome it will be is entirely down to you. Life on the desert planet is naturally harsh. The environment demands strength, endurance and the ability to survive and succeed on relatively few resources. Muscles have to justify every gram of their existence so there is no point having bulk when what you really need is strength. This is a workout worthy of a Sandworm Rider. Designed to build up core strength and dense muscle it's just the ticket for those whom Shai Hulud favors.

**Focus: Strength & Tone**

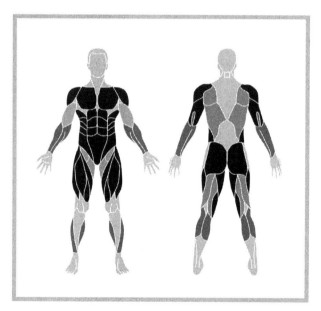

# FREMEN

DAREBEE WORKOUT © darebee.com

**LEVEL I** 3 sets **LEVEL II** 5 sets **LEVEL III** 7 sets **REST** up to 2 minutes

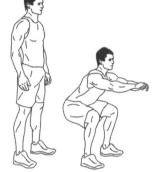

**10** squats

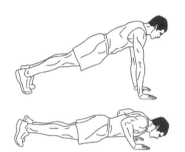

**5** push-ups

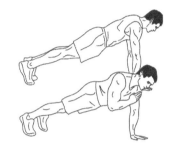

**10** shoulder taps

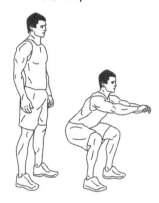

**10** squats

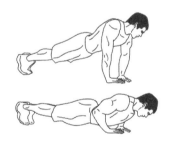

**5** close grip push-ups

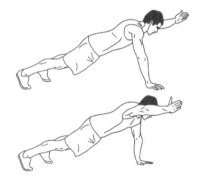

**10** plank arm raises

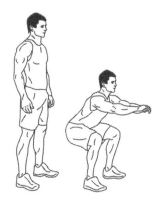

**10** squats

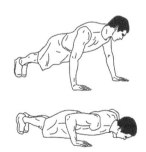

**5** wide grip push-ups

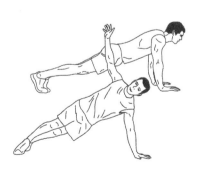

**10** planks w/ rotations

## 49 Frost

Even bad girls need to work out and our Frost routine, true to form, is a little bit of a killer. It's there to make sure that every part of your body can be called upon to play its role when needed. Now, stay frosty.

**Focus: High Burn**

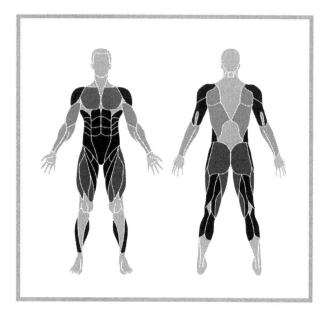

# FROST

## DAREBEE WORKOUT © darebee.com

**LEVEL I** 3 sets  **LEVEL II** 5 sets  **LEVEL III** 7 sets  **REST** up to 2 minutes

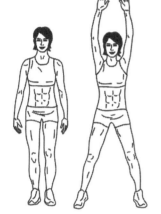

**20** jumping jacks

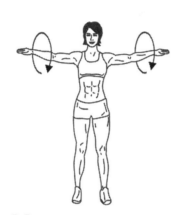

**20** raised arm circles

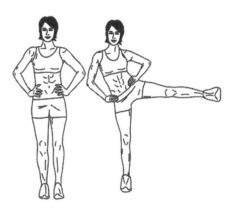

**20** side leg raises

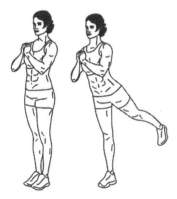

**20** low back kicks

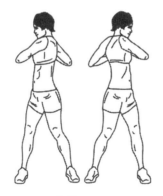

**20** twists

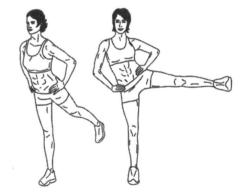

**20** back kick + side leg raise

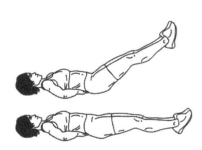

**10** leg raises

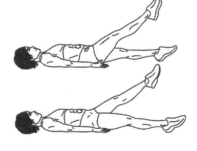

**10** flutter kicks

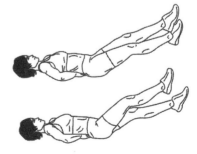

**10** scissors

## 50 Gamer

Whether on-screen or off it a Gamer needs to have some sound core stability and strength and the ability to control his body to the max. This workout is a pretty good place to start for those qualities.

**Focus: High Burn**

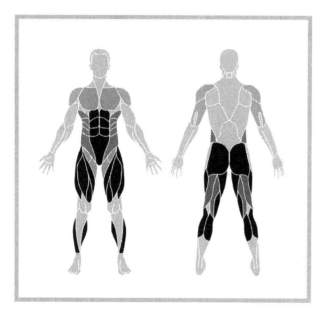

# GAMER

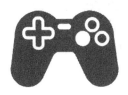

DAREBEE WORKOUT © darebee.com
**every respawn, construction or cinematic trailer**

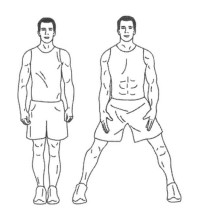

**20** half jacks

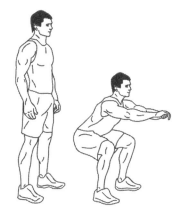

**10** squats

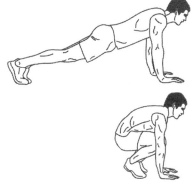

**10** plank jump-ins

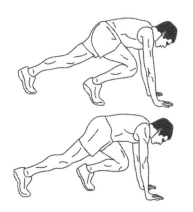

**20** climbers

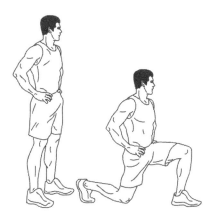

**10** lunges

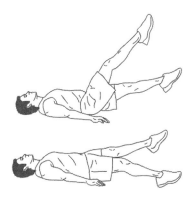

**10** flutter kicks

## 51 Gladiator

Gladiators were fierce people. To survive they required good core stability and strength followed by excellent ballistic movement capability. If you're ready to leap into the arena and battle to the death, for the glory of combat, then this workout is a good way to prepare.

**Focus: Strength & Tone**

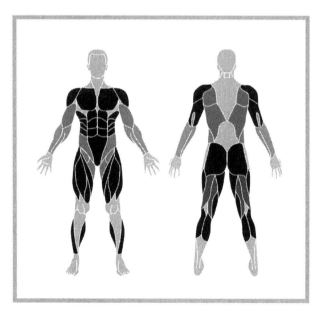

# GLADIATOR

DAREBEE WORKOUT © darebee.com

**LEVEL I** 3 sets **LEVEL II** 5 sets **LEVEL III** 7 sets **REST** up to 2 minutes

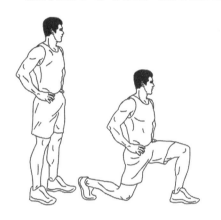

**40** lunges

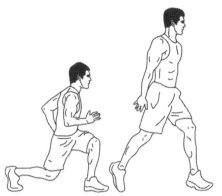

**20** jumping lunges

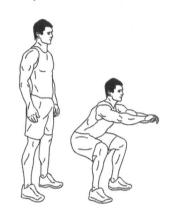

**20** squats

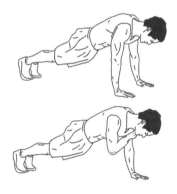

**20** shoulder taps

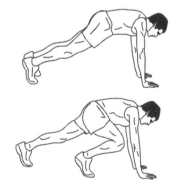

**40** slow climbers

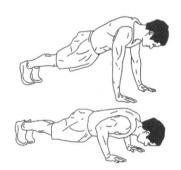

**10** push-ups

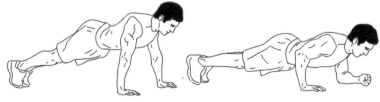

**10** up & down planks

## 52   Golem

If you're a mythical creature that's unstoppable you need the kind of basic strength and core power that renders you a force of nature. The Golem workout takes you back to basics for a reason. It really helps you take your core fitness to the level you need.

**Focus: Strength & Tone**

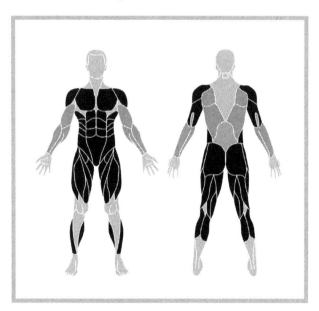

# GOLEM

DAREBEE WORKOUT © darebee.com

**LEVEL I** 3 sets **LEVEL II** 5 sets **LEVEL III** 7 sets **REST** up to 2 minutes

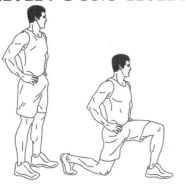

**20** lunges

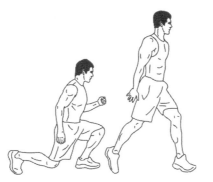

**10** jumping lunges

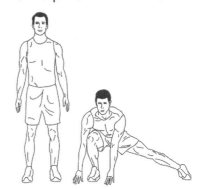

**10** side lunges

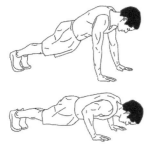

**10** push-ups

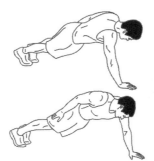

**10** thigh taps

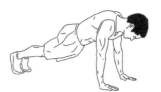

**10-count** plank

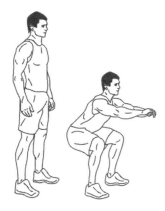

**20** squats

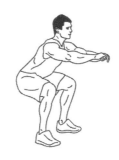

**10-count** squat hold

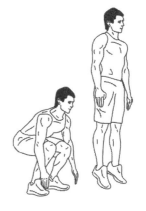

**10** jump squats

## 53 Gravity

To escape gravity you need dense muscles and strong bones and nothing gets muscles denser or bones stronger than a hyper-loaded floor workout.

Tips: There is little recovery time for each muscle group here so you need to make sure that your muscles get as much oxygen as possible by breathing in as deeply as possible at the recovery phase of each rep.

**Focus: Strength & Tone**

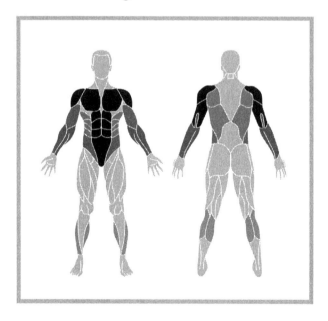

# GRAVITY

DAREBEE WORKOUT © darebee.com

**LEVEL I** 3 sets **LEVEL II** 4 sets **LEVEL III** 5 sets **REST** 2 minutes

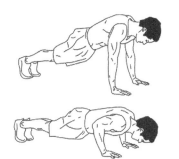

**4** push-ups

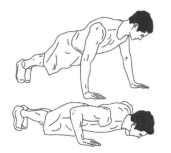

**4** wide grip

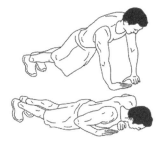

**2** close grip

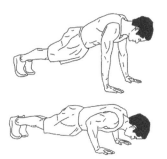

**4** push-ups

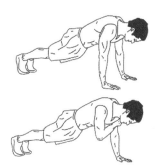

**4** shoulder taps

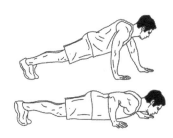

**2** staggered

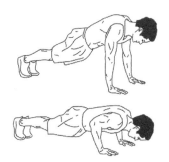

**4** push-ups

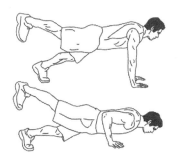

**4** raised leg

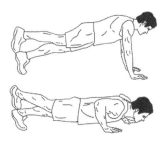

**2** stacked feet

## 54 Grounder

If you know your "The 100" genealogy you know a Grounder is naturally strong. A born survivor and a warrior by training. The Grounder workout is designed to help you develop the kind of solid strength you need to survive in a challenging environment. You just need to get through it, first.

Perfect for survivalists looking for that edgy training that'll push them up a level so they can become clan leaders. Plus, this is a heck of a workout for those days when you really want to blow some steam.

**Focus: Strength & Tone**

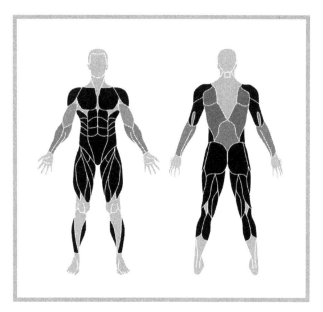

# GROUNDER

DAREBEE WORKOUT © darebee.com

**LEVEL I** 3 sets  **LEVEL II** 4 sets  **LEVEL III** 5 sets  **REST** up to 2 minutes

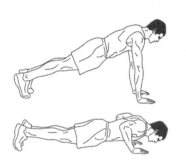

**10** push-ups

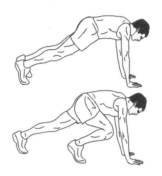

**20** slow climbers

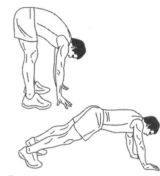

**10** plank walk-outs

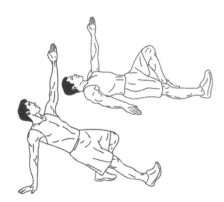

**10** get-ups

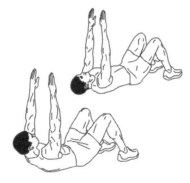

**20** high crunches

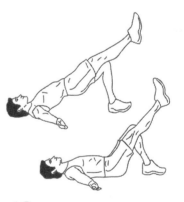

**10** one legged bridges

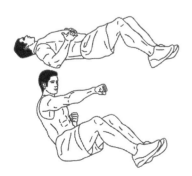

**10** sit-up punches

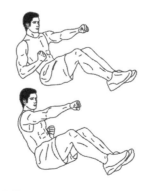

**20** sitting punches

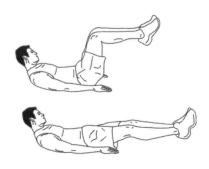

**10** crunch kicks

## 55 Guardian

You know just by the name of the workout that it's going to be a little challenging. A guardian is never needed unless there is something to 'guard' which means it is worth fighting over for, which means that you'd better shape up if you want to play this role. The Guardian workout will test every aspect of your fitness.

**Focus: Strength & Tone**

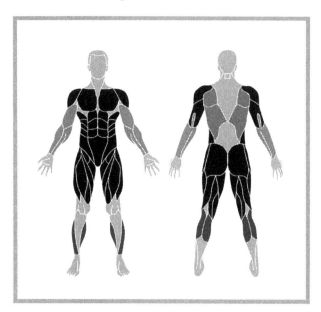

# GUARDIAN

## DAREBEE WORKOUT © darebee.com

**LEVEL I** 3 sets  **LEVEL II** 5 sets  **LEVEL III** 7 sets  **REST** up to 2 minutes

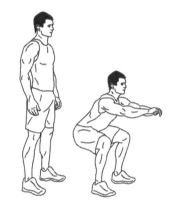

**10** squats

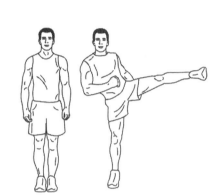

**20** side leg raises

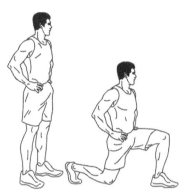

**10** lunges

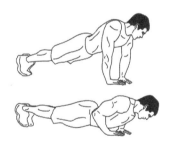

**5** close grip push-ups

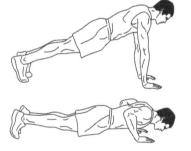

**10** push-ups

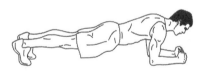

**10-count** elbow plank

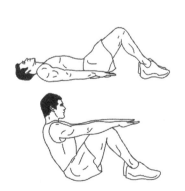

**10** sit-ups

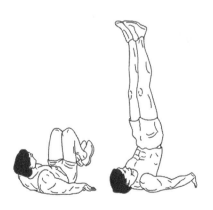

**10** butt-ups

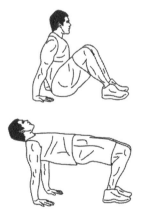

**10** full bridges

## 56 Guardsman

"I used to be an adventurer like you, but then I took an arrow in the knee" -
The Guardsman, Skyrim

Just because you had a little bad luck and took that arrow to the knee
doesn't mean your life has to be over. This is a workout for all those
suffering from knee problems, looking to change jobs from guarding the
city gates.

**Focus: Strength & Tone**

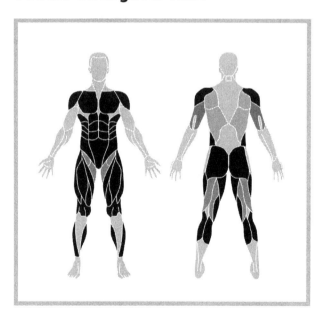

# GUARDSMAN

DAREBEE WORKOUT © darebee.com

**LEVEL I** 3 sets **LEVEL II** 5 sets **LEVEL III** 7 sets **REST** up to 2 minutes

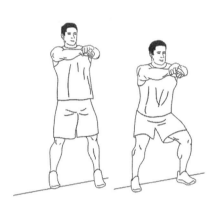

**20** wall half squats

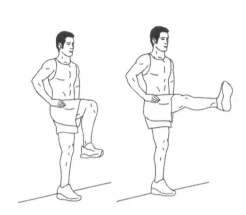

**20** slow front kicks

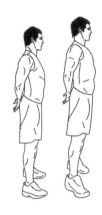

**20** calf raises

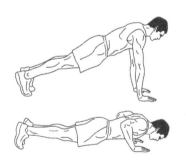

**10** push-ups

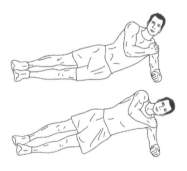

**10** side plank raises

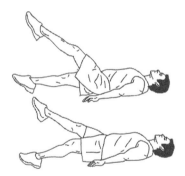

**20** flutter kicks

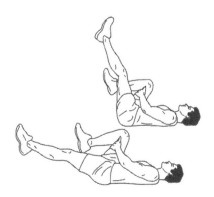

**10** lowering drills

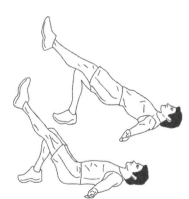

**10** single leg bridges

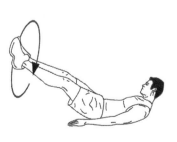

**10** raised leg circles

## 57  Hell's Circuit

Once in a while the moon turns red, the sky turns dark and there's a green glowing mist rising from the ground and that's exactly how you begin to perceive the world as you get past the 4-minute mark of the first set of Hell's Circuit. Designed to test the mettle of mortals, this a workout that transforms everyone who does it, even at Level I. The exercises appear deceptively easy but don't be fooled. Those who embark upon this little workout without feeling at least a little trepidation are destined for greatness.

**Focus:  High Burn, HIIT**

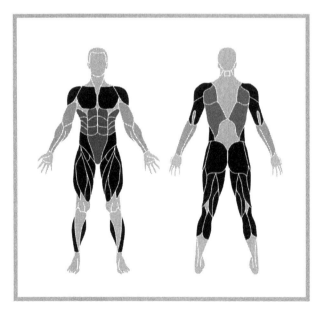

# Hell's Circuit

DAREBEE `HIIT` WORKOUT © darebee.com

**Level I** 3 rounds **Level II** 4 rounds **Level III** 5 rounds
1 minute each | 2 minutes rest between rounds

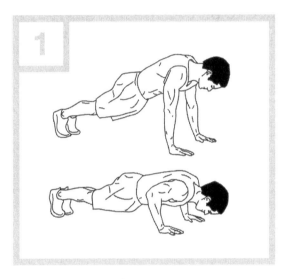

push-ups

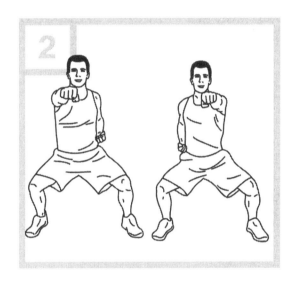

squat hold punches

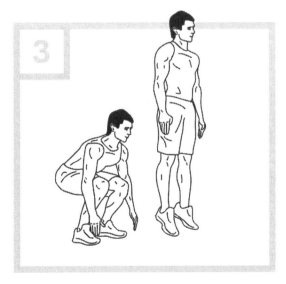

jump squats

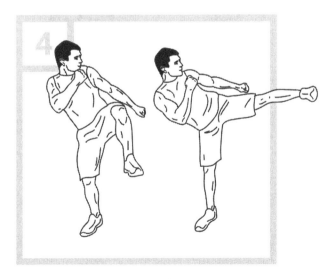

side kicks

## 58 Hercules

Even a demigod needs to do something to maintain his strength. This is the workout for those who are readying themselves to join the ranks of the Olympian pantheon and have to perform a few labours beforehand.

Tips: These are isometric exercise designed to pit one muscle group against another. When you perform them key to your success is having perfect form.

**Focus: Strength & Tone**

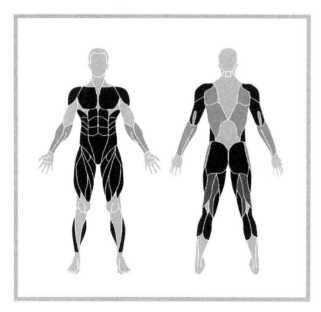

# HERCULES

DAREBEE WORKOUT © darebee.com

**LEVEL I** 3 sets  **LEVEL II** 5 sets  **LEVEL III** 7 sets  **REST** up to 2 minutes

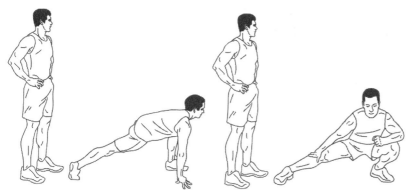
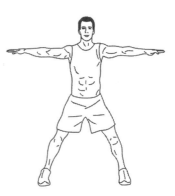

**20combos** lunge + deep side lunge          **40-count** star hold

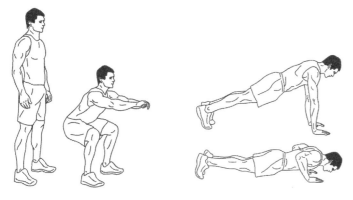
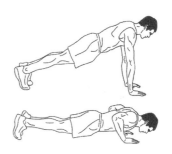

**20combos** squat + push-up          **20-count** push-up plank

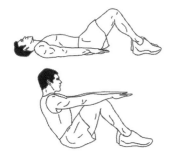
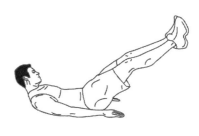

**20combos** sit-up + sitting twists          **40-count** raised leg hold

## 59    Homemade Back

Your back muscles are important not just because you need something sturdy to rest upon when you get to bed at night but also because they power all sorts of subtle body movements, from the power of punches thrown from the hip to how well you perform at pull ups and how strong your overhead throw is. The Homemade Back workout targets all the major muscle groups of your back without forgetting some other, equally important parts of your body.

**Focus: Strength & Tone**

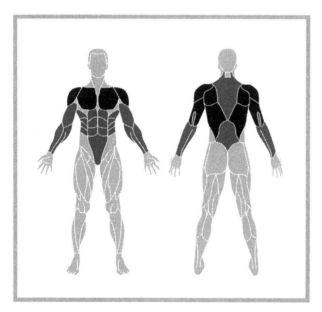

# HOMEMADE
# BACK

DAREBEE WORKOUT
© darebee.com
LEVEL I 3 sets
LEVEL II 5 sets
LEVEL III 7 sets
REST up to 2 minutes

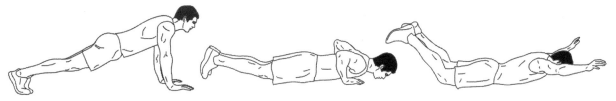

**10** diver push-ups

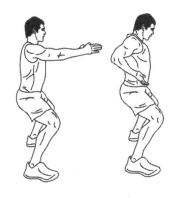

**20** half squat rows

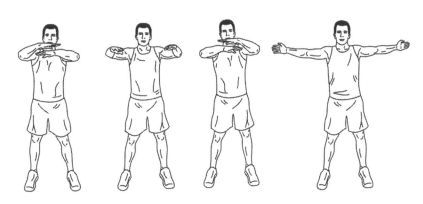

**20** double chest expansions

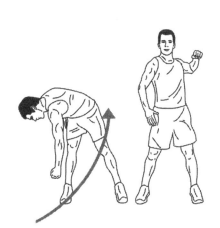

**20** lawnmowers

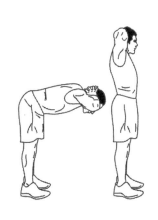

**20** forward bends

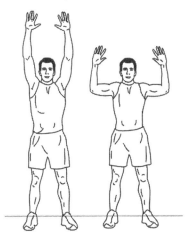

**20** wall arm slides

# 60    Hopper

Strong legs play a pivotal role to releasing the power of the upper body. This is a workout for those who really want to have legs of steel.

Tips: For maximum gains keep your body upright and centered over your feet during all hopping exercises.

**Focus: High Burn**

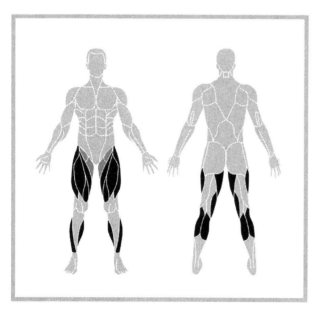

# HOPPER

DAREBEE WORKOUT © darebee.com

**LEVEL I** 3 sets **LEVEL II** 5 sets **LEVEL III** 7 sets **REST** up to 2 minutes
20 seconds each exercise | no rest between exercises

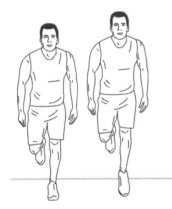

hop on one leg

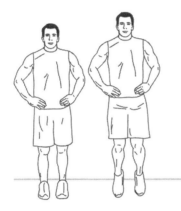

hop on
both legs

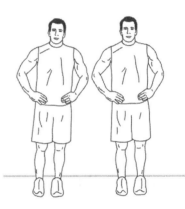

hop from
side to side
on both legs

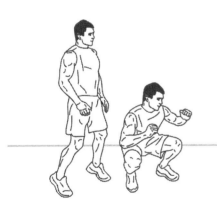

double hop
& squat

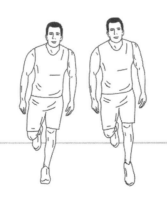

hop from
side to side
on one leg

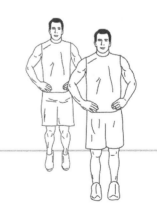

hop back
& forward
on both legs

## 61 Huntress

In ancient Greek mythology, Diana was the goddess of the hunt and she was fit enough to run with her hounds and take down stags. The Huntress workout may not quite put you in the same league but you will definitely notice a change if you keep it up for a while. It is a whole body challenge that also pushes against the limits of your circulatory and breathing systems.

**Focus: High Burn**

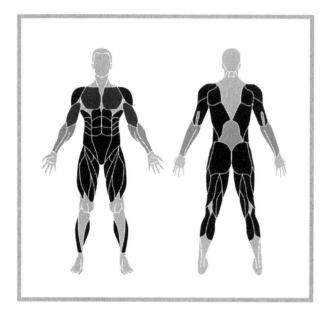

# HUNTRESS

DAREBEE WORKOUT © darebee.com

**LEVEL I** 3 sets  **LEVEL II** 5 sets  **LEVEL III** 7 sets  **REST** up to 2 minutes

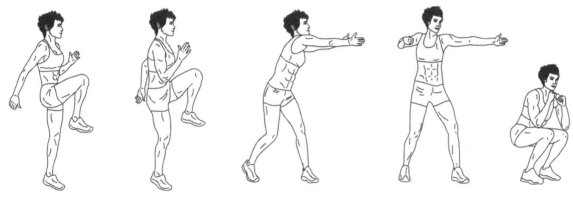

**5combos:**   **10** high knees  +  **2** archers  +  **2** squats

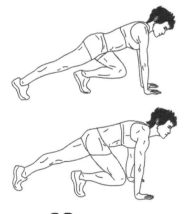

**20** climbers

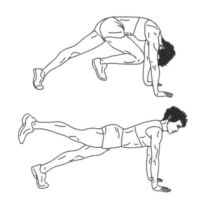

**10** knee-in kick backs

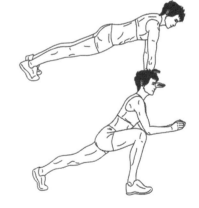

**10** plank-into-lunges

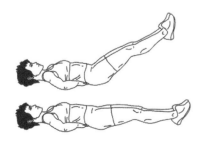

**10** leg raises

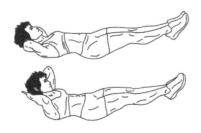

**10** raised legs crunches

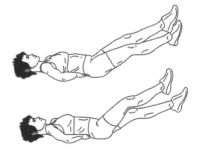

**10** scissors

## 62　Infinity

While you may never, ever be able to go beyond infinity you will be able to feel the journey as you put your body through its paces. The Infinity workout is designed to help you free your body as you strengthen all the muscles you need to help your movements flow.

**Focus: High Burn**

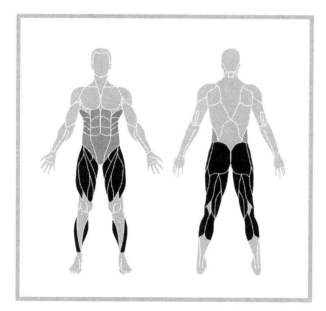

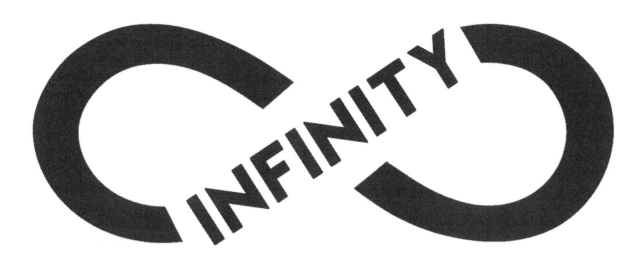

# DAREBEE WORKOUT © darebee.com

**LEVEL I** 3 sets **LEVEL II** 5 sets **LEVEL III** 7 sets **REST** up to 2 minutes

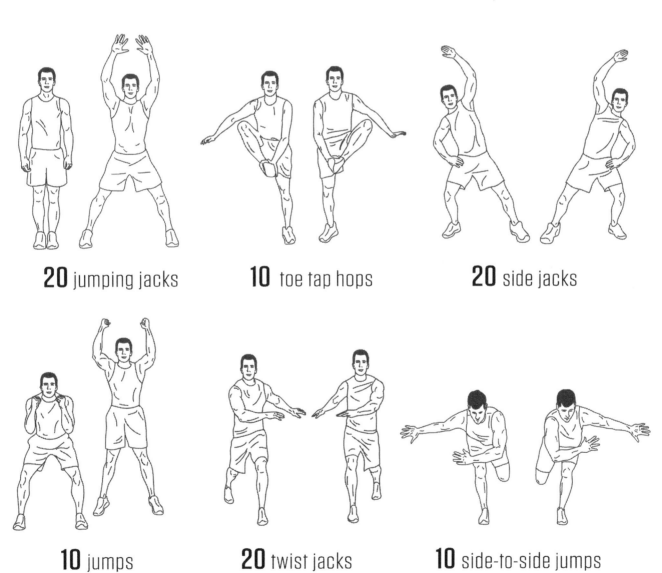

**20** jumping jacks

**10** toe tap hops

**20** side jacks

**10** jumps

**20** twist jacks

**10** side-to-side jumps

## 63   Ivy

A body does not get strong and lithe without work. It takes sustained work that targets many muscle groups to get the kind of results that turn heads and the Ivy workout is designed to make a lot of muscle groups work together for faster results. Not that time is the issue here. Effectiveness is and the results speak for themselves. This is a workout that simply asks you to develop power and strength with grace.

**Focus: Strength & Tone**

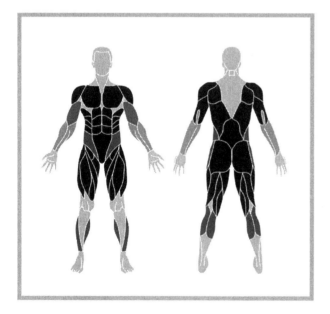

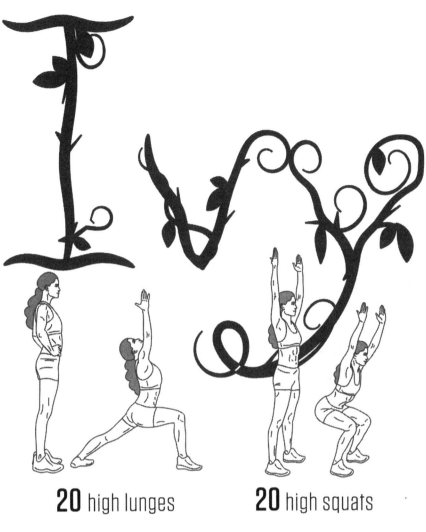

DAREBEE WORKOUT
© darebee.com
**LEVEL I** 3 sets
**LEVEL II** 5 sets
**LEVEL III** 7 sets
**REST** up to 2 minutes

**20** high lunges

**20** high squats

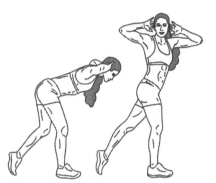

**20** deadlift twists

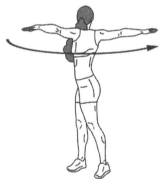

**20** rotations

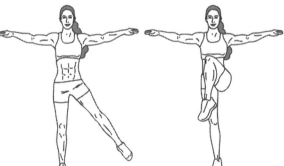

**20** leg swing + knee up

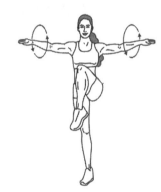

**20** arm rotations

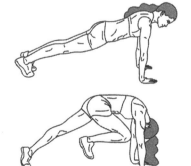

**10** plank knee-ins

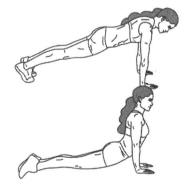

**10** upward dog

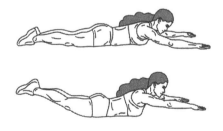

**10** superman stretches

## 64 Jacks Pyramid

Some workouts are just designed to put emphasis on "work". Without work there can be no change. Without change there can be no improvement. And improvement there shall be with the Jacks Pyramid workout. 'Nuff said.

Make it harder: Reduce rest time between sets to just 60 seconds it will challenge your aerobic performance and muscle recovery times.

**Focus: High Burn**

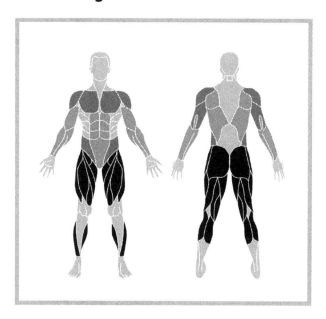

# JACKS PYRAMID

DAREBEE WORKOUT © darebee.com

**LEVEL I** 3 sets **LEVEL II** 5 sets **LEVEL III** 7 sets **REST** up to 2 minutes

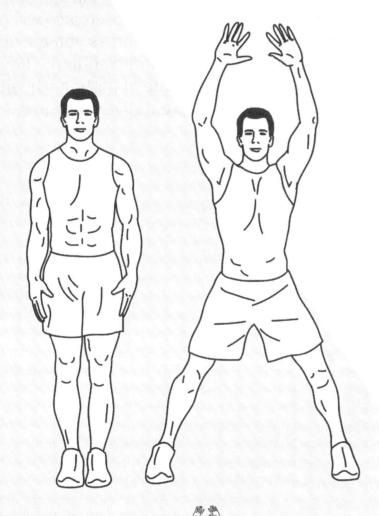

**10** jumping jacks

10-count rest

**15** jumping jacks

10-count rest

**20** jumping jacks

10-count rest

**25** jumping jacks

10-count rest

**20** jumping jacks

10-count rest

**15** jumping jacks

10-count rest

**10** jumping jacks

**LOW IMPACT ALTERNATIVE STEP JACKS**

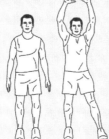

## 65 Knee Workout

Knees take a pounding even before an arrow happens to find them. Because the knee is a hinge type synovial joint it presents a level of complexity not seen in other joints. Conditioning of the surrounding muscles is crucial in achieving joint stability and preventing injury. If you have been unlucky enough to have been injured here, the exercises will help add to the speed of rehabilitation of the knee joint (as long as you are not at one of the stages of injury that require operational intervention). The exercises here are designed to help maintain the range of motion a healthy knee joint is capable of. They can also work as preventative measures, taken to avoid sustaining knee injuries.

**Focus: Stretching**

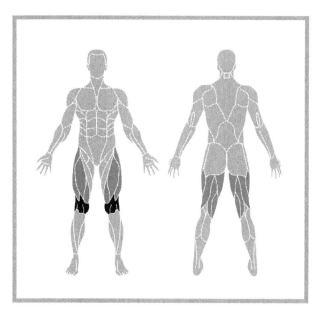

# KNEE

REHAB WORKOUT
© darebee.com
**LEVEL I** 3 sets
**LEVEL II** 5 sets
**LEVEL III** 7 sets
**REST** up to 2 minutes

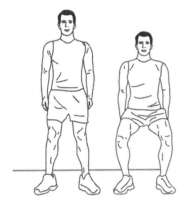

**10** wall half squats

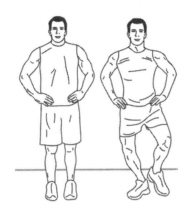

**10** wide single leg squats

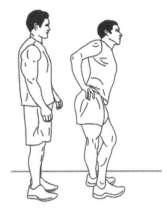

**30sec** cross leg side tilts

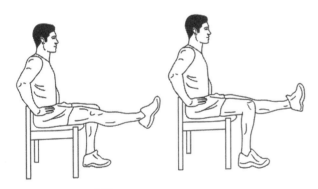

**10** leg raises

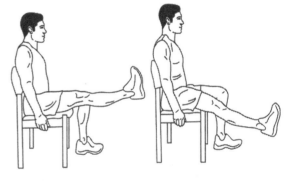

**20** raised leg swings

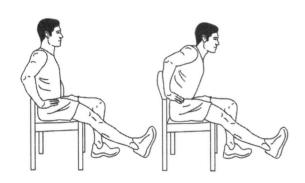

**30sec** hamstring stretch

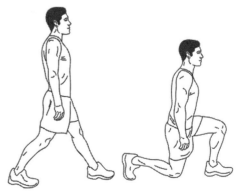

**10** split squats

# 66 Leg Day

Legs are what you need to use when you want to run (from zombies, werewolves and vampires, for example) and they're also kinda useful in everyday life because we still walk to get to places. This is a workout to help you make them strong and capable of performing at will.

**Focus: Strength & Tone**

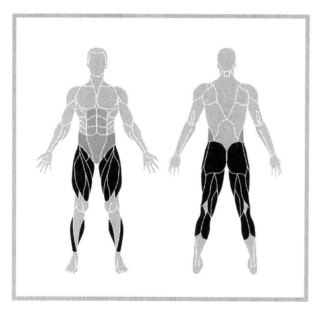

# Leg Day

DAREBEE WORKOUT © darebee.com

**LEVEL I** 3 sets **LEVEL II** 4 sets **LEVEL III** 5 sets **REST** up to 2 minutes

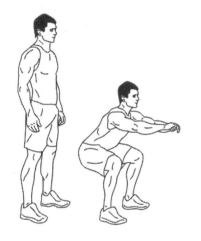

**40** squats

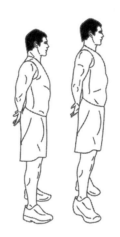

**20** calf raises

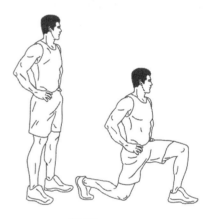

**20** lunges

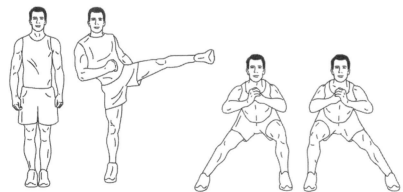

**20** side leg raises

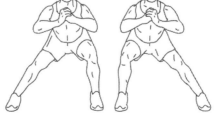

**20** side-to-side lunges

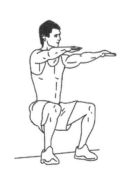

**20-count** wall-sit

## 67 Loop

If you want to have the energy of the Energizer Bunny then this workout is going to give you the right kind of burn. Each exercise flows into the next one so you're working out non-stop at a steady pace until you, well ... drop or the allotted time runs out (whichever one comes first).

Tip:Pace is key here. Start too fast and you will burn out before the time is up. Go too slow and you will end up with more fuel in the tank than you really need. So find the pace you think you can maintain and ignore the burn. It's good for you.

**Focus: Strength & Tone**

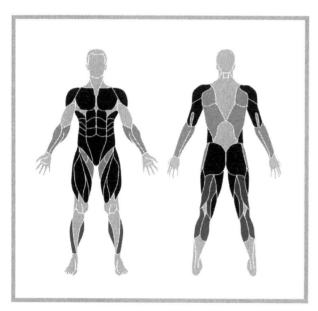

# LOOP

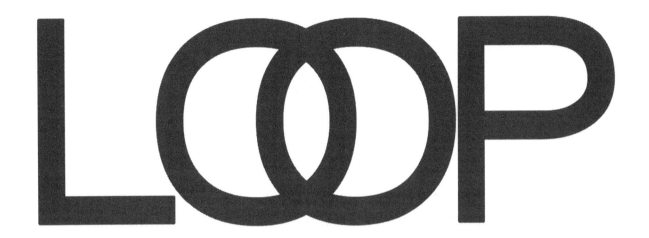

DAREBEE WORKOUT © darebee.com
set the timer for **10 minutes** repeat the circuit until the time is up
**LEVEL I** 6 reps   **LEVEL II** 10 reps   **LEVEL III** 20 reps

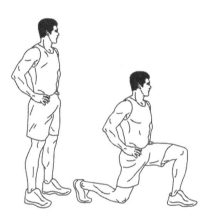

lunges

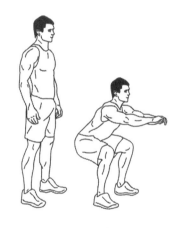

squats

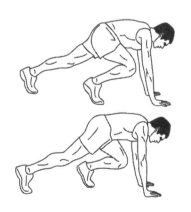

climbers

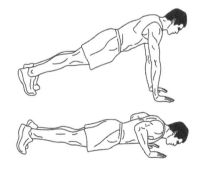

push-ups

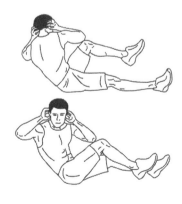

knee-to-elbow crunches

## 68 Lower Back

Instructions: Repeat each move one after the other with no rest in between until the set is done, rest up to 2 minutes and repeat the whole set again, 3 times in total.

Hold the stretch for one deep breath and return to the starting position. Repeat each move with no rest in between until the set is done.

**Focus: Stretching**

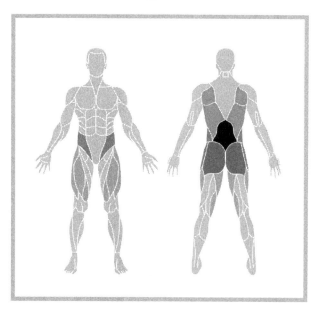

# LOWER BACK

REHAB WORKOUT
© darebee.com
**3 sets** | 2 minutes rest

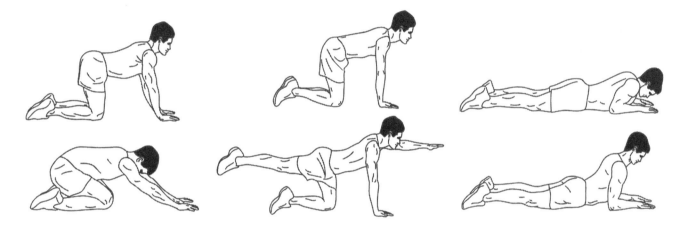

**10** bottom to heels stretch   **10** opposite arm / leg raises   **10** back extensions

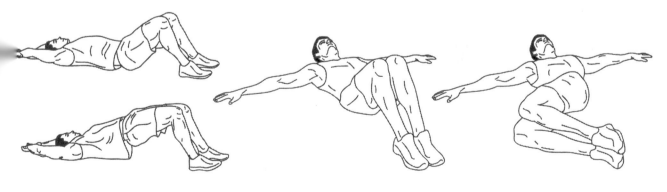

**10** bridges   **10** knee rolls

## 69    Make me a Sandwich

In order to qualify for your sandwich you really need to earn it and this is the workout that makes sure you do just that. This is a high-burn, lower body workout that'll have you feeling the benefits in no time at all. Earn your sandwich!

Tips: If you want to develop explosiveness in your movements this workout helps you to do just that. Tackle each exercise at 100% output to build lean, fast twitch fiber muscle.

Earn your sandwich!

**Focus: High Burn**

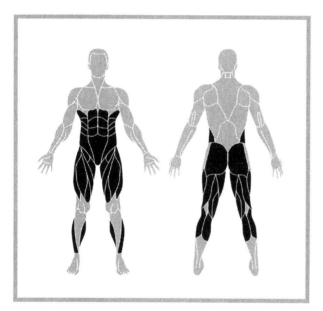

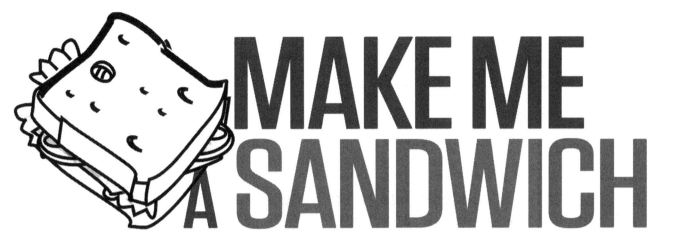

# MAKE ME A SANDWICH

DAREBEE WORKOUT © darebee.com

**LEVEL I** 3 sets **LEVEL II** 5 sets **LEVEL III** 7 sets **REST** up to 2 minutes

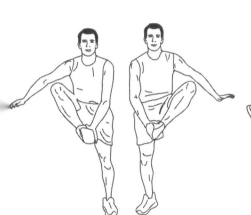

**20** toe tap jumps

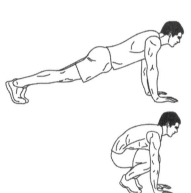

**20** plank jump-ins

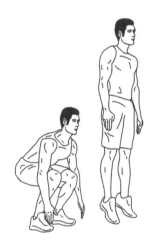

**5** jump squats

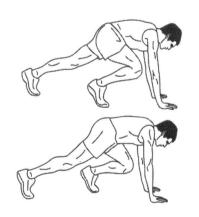

**20** climbers

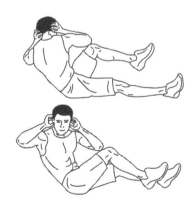

**20** knee-to-elbow crunches

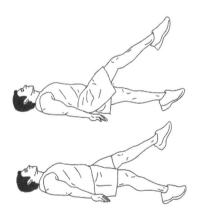

**20** flutter kicks

## 70 Mass Blast

Developed to help you storm hills and race up mountains this is the workout for those looking to unlock all the power of their lower body.

Tips: Strength requires repetition and getting through the set. So irrespective of speed and irrespective of burn, bite the bullet and get this baby done.

**Focus:  High Burn, HIIT**

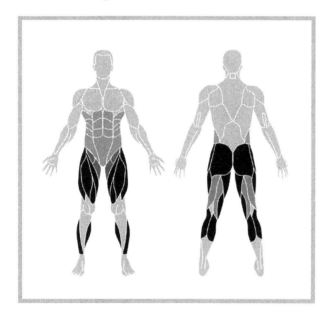

# MASS BLAST

DAREBEE `HIIT` WORKOUT © darebee.com

**Level I**  5 rounds   **Level II**  10 rounds   **Level III**  15 rounds
1 minute rest between rounds

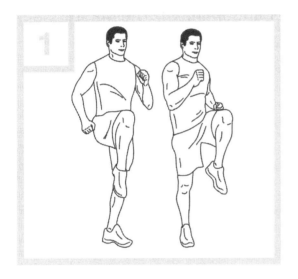

**15sec** high knees

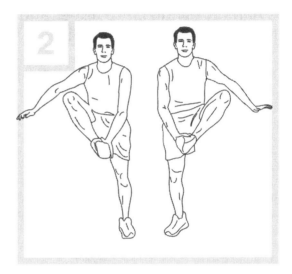

**15sec** toe tap hops

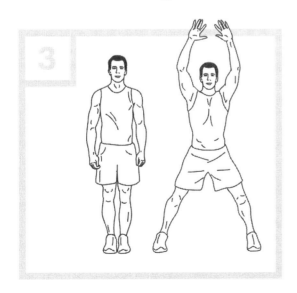

**15sec** jumping jacks

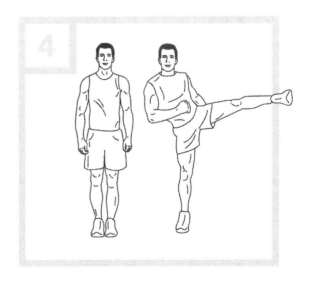

**15sec** side leg raises

## 71 Master Pack

When you're talking six-pack you're really talking about more muscle groups than one. The abdominals are made up of four distinct muscle groups: the Transverse Abdominis (also called core), the External Abdominal Obliques, the Internal Abdominal Obliques, the Rectus Abdominis (which also happen to be handily divided into upper and lower abdominals). The Master Pack workout takes care of them all.

**Focus: Abs**

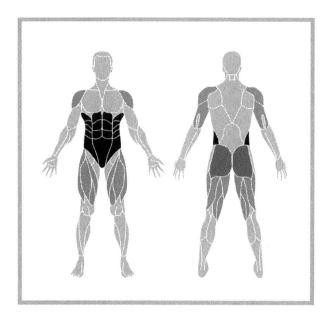

# Master Pack

DAREBEE WORKOUT © darebee.com

**LEVEL I** 3 sets **LEVEL II** 4 sets **LEVEL III** 5 sets **REST** up to 2 minutes

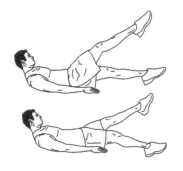

**20** flutter kicks

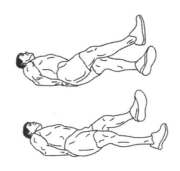

**20** scissors

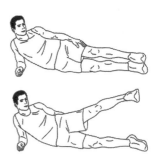

**20** side leg raises

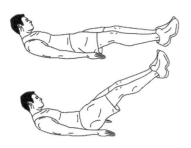

**10** leg raises

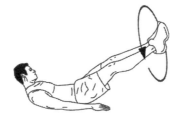

**10** raised leg circles

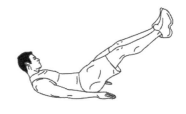

**20sec** raised leg hold

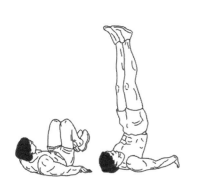

**10** butt-ups

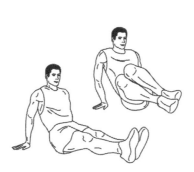

**10** knee-in & twist

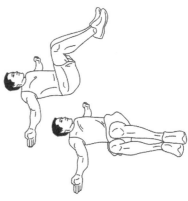

**10** half wipers

# 72 Maximus

Get ready to command the Legions of the North by prepping yourself with the Maximus workout. Not only will your body feel ready for combat but should you find yourself in a field of dust, with the crowd around you, a gladius in one hand, do not be troubled, for you are now a Gladiator.

**Focus: Strength & Tone**

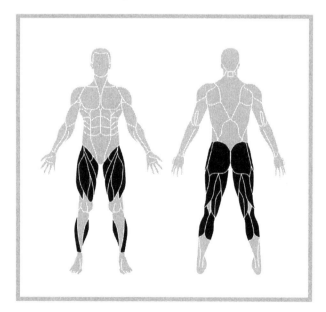

# maXimus

DAREBEE WORKOUT © darebee.com

**LEVEL I** 3 sets **LEVEL II** 4 sets **LEVEL III** 5 sets **REST** up to 2 minutes

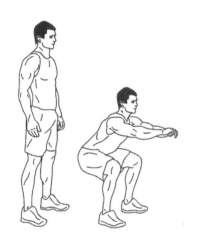

**20** squats

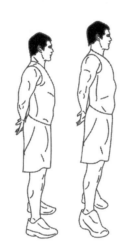

**20** calf raises

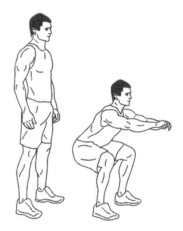

**20** squats

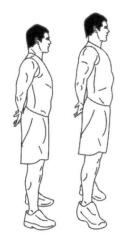

**20** calf raises

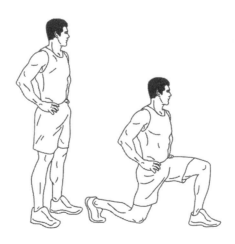

**40** lunges

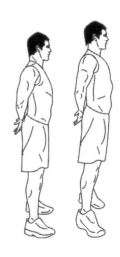

**20** calf raises

# 73 Movie Night

You know that feeling when all you want to do is sit at home watching something on TV? The world outside has ceased to exist but that doesn't mean that your drive for fitness needs to go bye-bye. Quite the opposite in fact. Here's a chance to turn that sofa into your playground making the night-in movie your fitness aid. If you want to have your cake and eat it, this is the perfect way to start. So indulge, watch that film and chill at home and don't forget to make your reps count.

Tips: This is a great tendon-strengthening, low-key workout. If you really want to test yourself cut down the rest time between sets to 30 seconds and get ready to feel some serious burn in your tendons.

**Focus: High Burn**

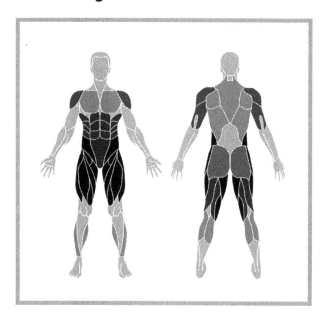

# movie night

DAREBEE WORKOUT © darebee.com

Repeat 3 times | up to 2 minutes rest between sets

**or every 20 minutes during a movie**

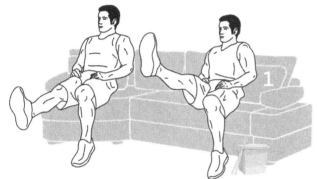

**20** leg swings

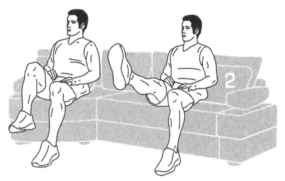

**20** front snap kicks

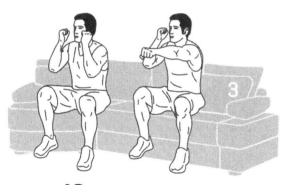

**40** punches

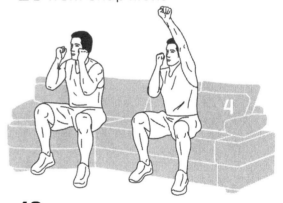

**40** overhead punches

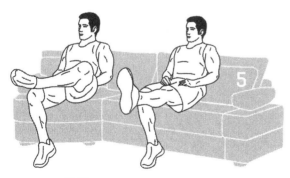

**20** knee taps

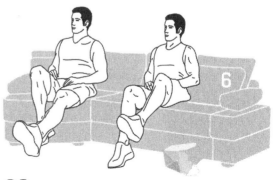

**20** air bike crunches

## 74 Neck Workout

Neck pain is one of the most common complaints of our digitally-enhanced society. Time spent in front of screens or looking at our devices, insufficient focus on neck muscles during our workouts and too little time to spend on this muscle group in general contribute to frequent complaints. The Neck Pain and Tension Relief workout remedies all those problems. It can be performed as a warm-up, before exercise or as a total stress reliever at the end of the day.

**Focus: Stretching**

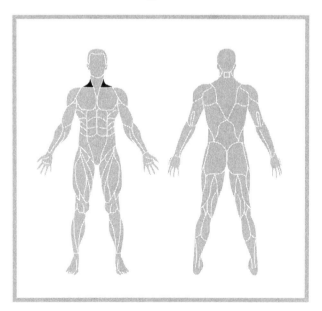

# NECK

DAREBEE WORKOUT
© darebee.com
**3 sets** | 2 minutes rest

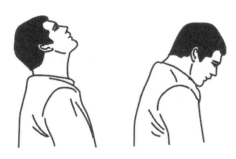

**10** back and forth tilts

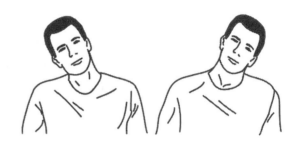

**10** side-to-side tilts

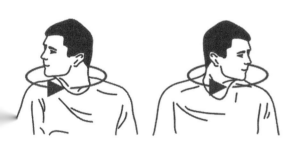

**10** neck rotations

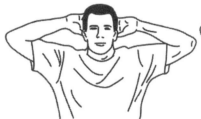

**10-count** press

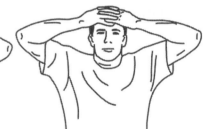

**10-count** press

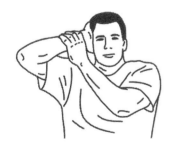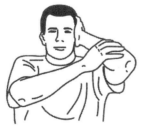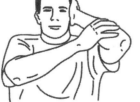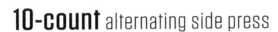

**10-count** alternating side press

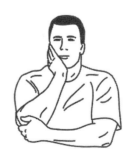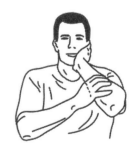

**10-count** alternating chin press

## 75 Ninja

The ninja, legendary assassins of the night were possessed of great lower body strength and agility. This is a workout that aims at the muscle groups that give you both these qualities.

Tips: When performing side leg raises lean towards the leg you raise rather than leaning away from it. This increases the tension on your lateral abdominals and promotes greater core strength and stability.

**Focus: High Burn**

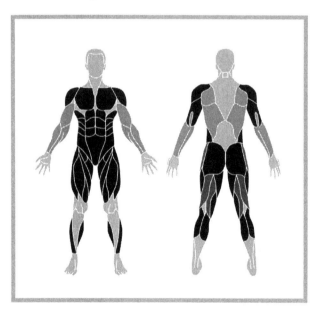

# NINJA

SILENT WORKOUT BY DAREBEE © darebee.com

**LEVEL I** 3 sets **LEVEL II** 5 sets **LEVEL III** 7 sets **REST** up to 2 minutes

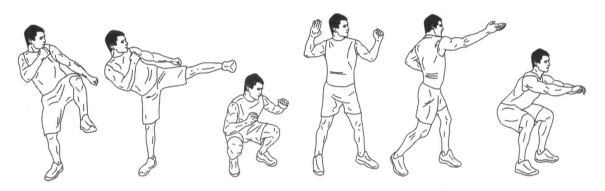

**40** side kicks   **20 combos** squat + knife hand strike   **20-count** squat hold

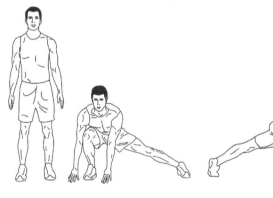

**10** side lunges

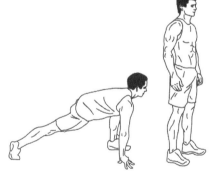

**10** reverse deep lunges

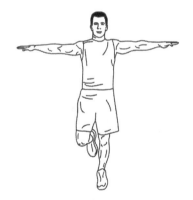

**20-count** one leg stand

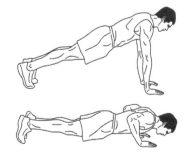

**10** push-ups

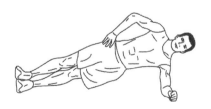

**20-count** side elbow plank

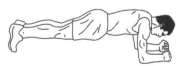

**20-count** elbow plank

## 76 Odin

Valhalla is a place where the gods don't just drink and revel but also train and fight. The Wrath of Odin workout is for those ready to prepare for that kind of 'revel' by punishing their body. Good for the soul and probably the closest you get to feeling like a Norse god.

Make it harder. Clear the floor by at least a foot when performing jump squats.

**Focus: High Burn**

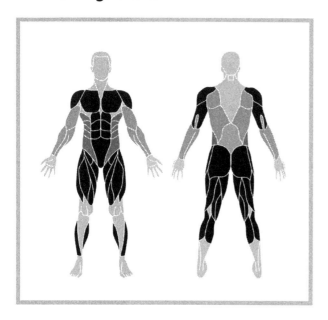

# THE WRATH OF
# ODIN

DAREBEE WORKOUT © darebee.com

**LEVEL I** 3 sets **LEVEL II** 5 sets **LEVEL III** 7 sets **REST** up to 2 minutes

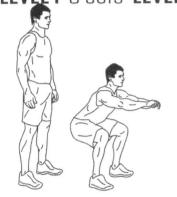 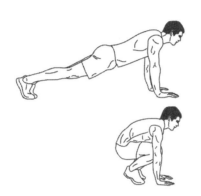 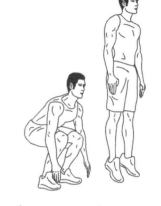

**20combos** squat + plank jump-in + jump squat

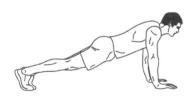 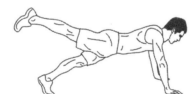 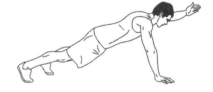

**10-count each** plank + raised leg plank + raised arm plank

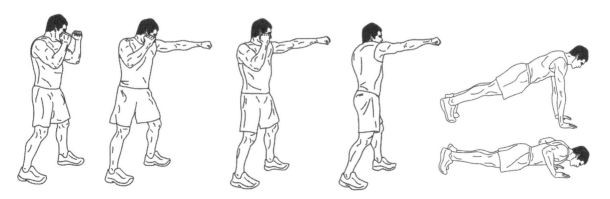

**20combos** jab + jab + cross + push-up

## 77 Office

Just because you're at the office does not mean you can't workout. This is the kind of exercise routine that can be carried out anywhere you have a little space and some privacy.

Tips: None of this need be done fast. You are, after all, at the office. But do them in a focused way and they help you work out every single muscle group of your body.

**Focus: Strength & Tone**

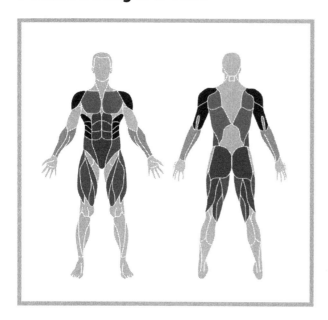

# office

DAREBEE WORKOUT © darebee.com

**LEVEL I** 3 sets  **LEVEL II** 5 sets  **LEVEL III** 7 sets  **REST** up to 2 minutes

**20** chair squats

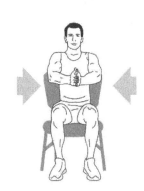

**20** chest squeezes

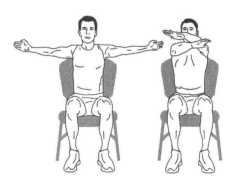

**40** criss-cross arms

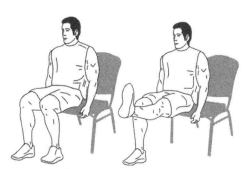

**40** leg extensions

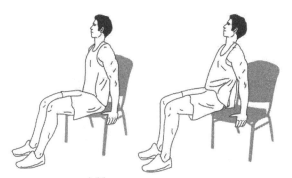

**10** chair body lifts

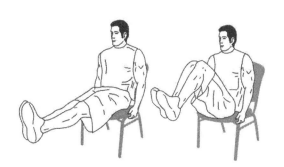

**10** knee pull-ins

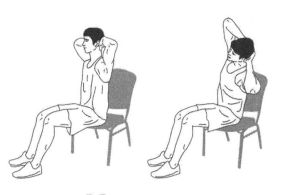

**20** oblique bends

## 78 Parkour

Your body is always the means through which you express your persona philosophy. Nowhere is this more evident perhaps than when it comes to Free Running or Parkour. Here mind meets body meets the physical world in the purest sense of the word. You need to let go of your fears, free your mind and embrace your environment in ways that are are truly liberating. Even if you're not going to go and try this on your nearest rooftop, having a go at the park is enough to change the way you perceive the world you live in. It also totally changes the relationship you have with your body. In order to throw it around and have it do wild things you need to have total trust in your physical abilities. And trust, starts right here. Right now. With this.

**Focus: Strength & Tone**

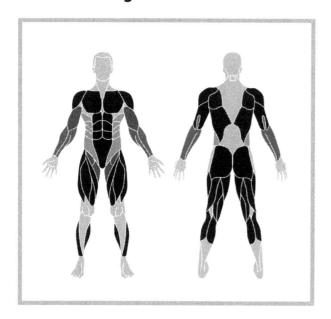

## basics

# parkour

### DAREBEE WORKOUT © darebee.com

**LEVEL I** 3 sets **LEVEL II** 5 sets **LEVEL III** 7 sets **REST** up to 2 minutes

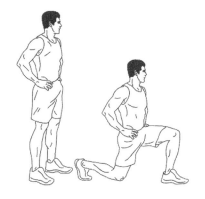

**10** lunges

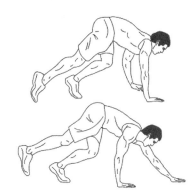

**10-count** bear crawl

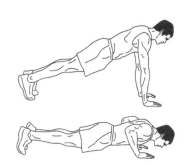

**10** push-ups

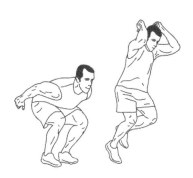

**10** broad jumps

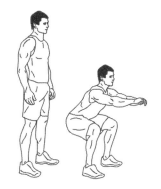

**20** squats

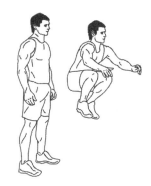

**10** jump knee-tucks

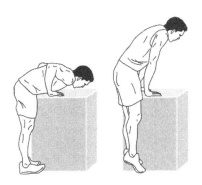

**10** wall dips

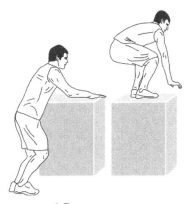

**10** plant plyos

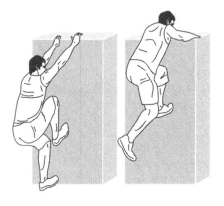

**10** wall climbers

## 79   Park Workout

A walk in the park will never be better for you than when you also get some exercise along with your hefty dose of the sunshine and fresh air. The A Walk in a Park workout is perfect for productively filling in your Summer downtime, working up a little sweat and feeling like you've escaped to nature, at least for a while. The workout is light but then again you're walking, it's a park and it should be Summer, or at the very least a sunny day. Enjoy it.

Make it harder. Go faster. Try to beat your own time for each set. Be warned. You will get stares.

**Focus: High Burn**

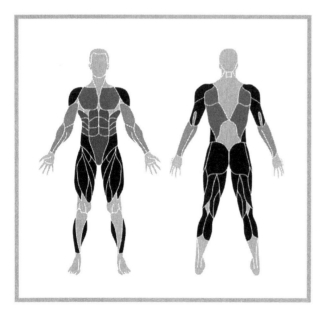

# a walk in a Park

DAREBEE WORKOUT © darebee.com

**20 reps each** | 5 sets in total

up to 2 minutes rest between sets

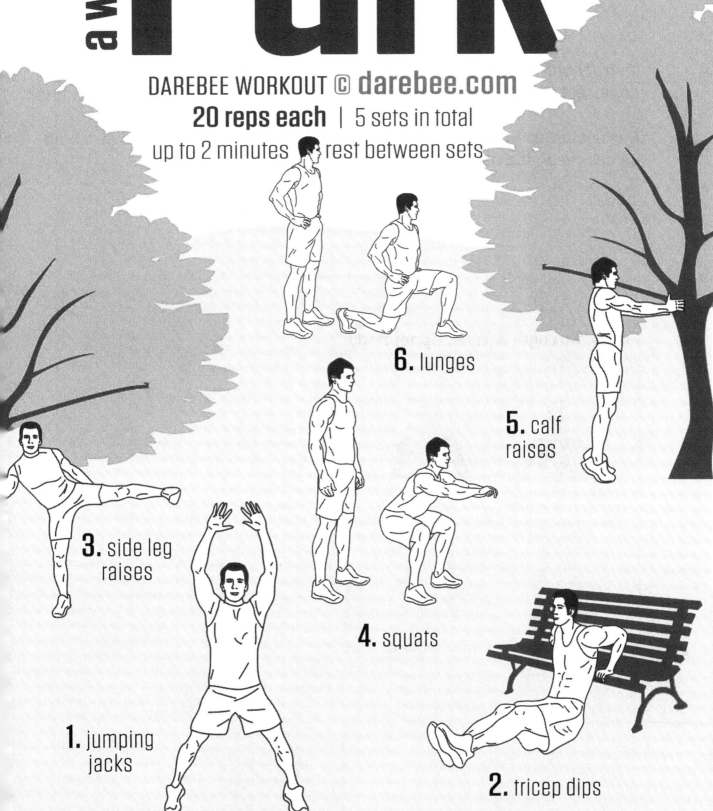

**6.** lunges

**5.** calf raises

**3.** side leg raises

**4.** squats

**1.** jumping jacks

**2.** tricep dips

## 80 Power 15

Instructions: Repeat each move with no rest in between until the set is done, rest up to 60 seconds and repeat the whole set again, 3 times in total.

Make it better: Perform arm raises, raised arm circles and raised arm hold balancing on the balls of your feet for a challenge to your core.

**Focus: Strength & Tone, Upper Body**

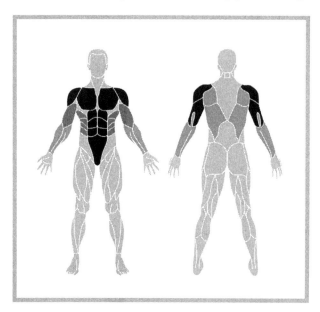

# Power 15

DAREBEE WORKOUT © darebee.com

3 sets | 60 seconds rest between sets
Keep your arms up between arm circles to arm hold

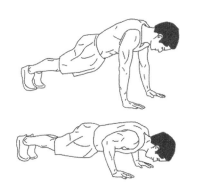

**to failure** push-ups

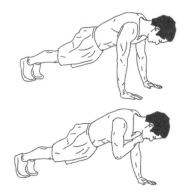

**20** shoulder taps

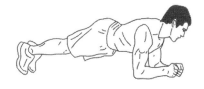

**20sec** elbow plank

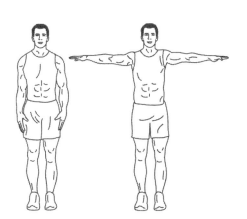

**20** arm raises

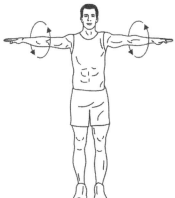

**20** raised arm circles

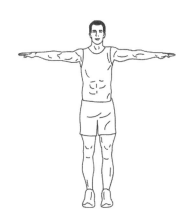

**20sec** raised arm hold

| 81 | Pie |
|---|---|

Nothing wrong with some pie as long as you get to earn it first. This is the workout that helps you do just that. Go and get ready to save the world, earn yourself some pie.

Tips: When you perform planks with rotations make sure that you turn your body completely sideways. Lightly tense your lower abs by exhaling to help stabilise the abdominal muscles and bring the lower abs into play.

**Focus: High Burn**

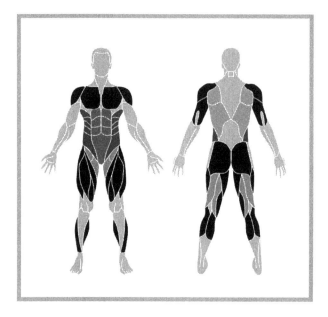

# BRING ME SOME PIE

DAREBEE WORKOUT © darebee.com

**LEVEL I** 3 sets **LEVEL II** 5 sets **LEVEL III** 7 sets **REST** up to 2 minutes

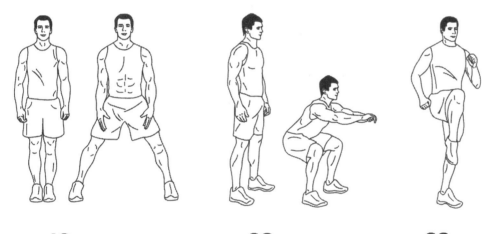

**40** half jacks          **20** squats          **20** high knees

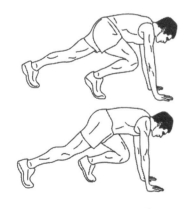          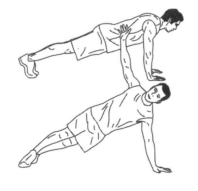          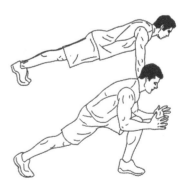

**20** climbers          **10** planks with rotations          **10** push-up into lunges

## 82    Pillow Fight

You know when you use to have pillow fights when you were a kid because you thought they were cool and your parents used to step in and break them up and tell you they weren't? Well, guess what? You were right and your parents were wrong. A good ol' fashioned pillow fight is the coolest way we know to get the blood flowing through your body, work some great muscle groups and, even, work up some sweat. This workout should be taken straight to your parents with an "I told you so" note. One small not of caution, should you get over-enthusiastic you may want to rethink the decor of the room you're exercising in. We are speaking from experience when we say that vases and small porcelain figurines do not enjoy a natural lifespan with this exercise routine in action around them.

**Focus: High Burn**

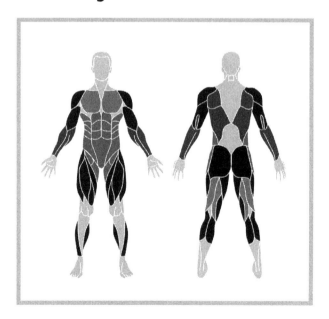

# pillow fight

DAREBEE WORKOUT © darebee.com

repeat 5 times | up to 2 minute rest between sets

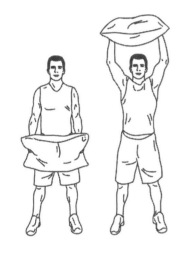

**20** pillow presses

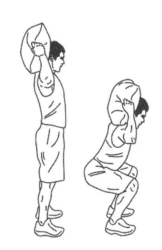

**10** pillow squats

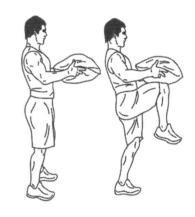

**10** pillow high knees

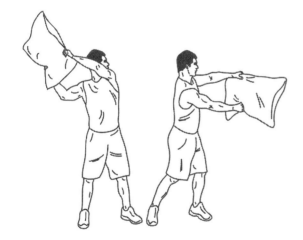

**20** pillow strikes

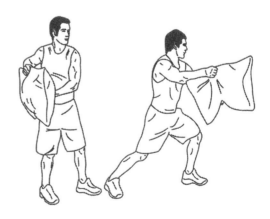

**20** pillow lunges

## 83 Playground

When you were a kid the playground was where you worked out your Spiderman and Tarzan fantasies. It was the place where your body encountered obstacles and met forces, like gravity. Being a kid is a state of mind. Rediscover the magic and get fitter in the process with the Playground workout. Commandeer the nearest one to you and get ready to feel the benefits of peeling back time. Just remember that this time round there are no excuses for not sharing your space. You really do know better.

**Focus: Strength & Tone**

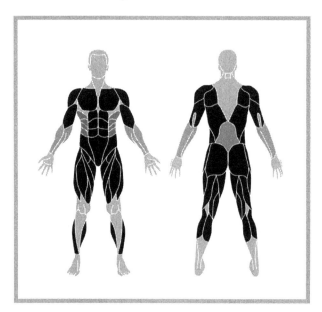

# PlayGround

DAREBEE WORKOUT © darebee.com

**LEVEL I** 3 sets **LEVEL II** 5 sets **LEVEL III** 7 sets **REST** up to 2 minutes

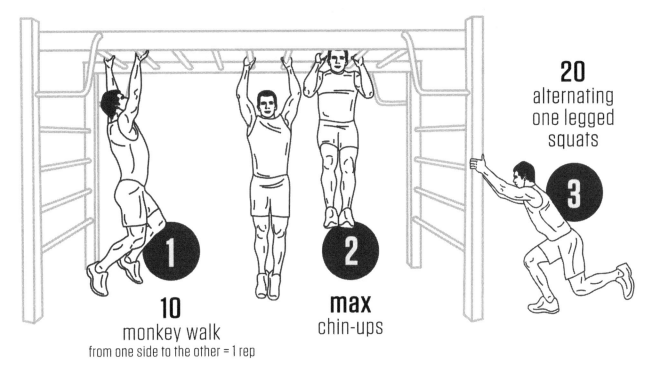

**20** alternating one legged squats **3**

**10** monkey walk
from one side to the other = 1 rep

**max** chin-ups

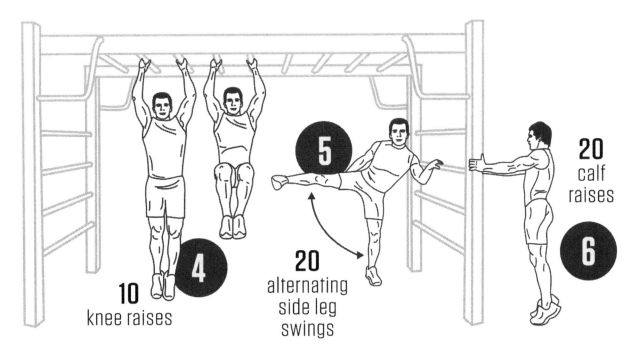

**20** alternating side leg swings

**20** calf raises **6**

**10** knee raises

## 84   Power Up

This is an aerobic workout that develops strength, flexibility and balance. Do it every time you want to top up your abilities in these three areas.

Tips: When performing lunge kicks keep your body as straight as possible and bring your foot up to your hand, not your hand to your foot.

**Focus: High Burn**

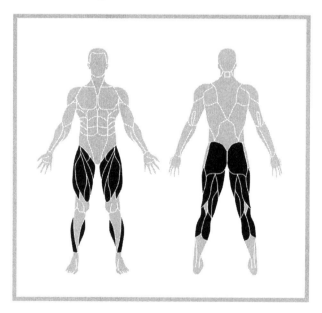

# POWER UP

DAREBEE WORKOUT © darebee.com

**LEVEL I** 3 sets  **LEVEL II** 5 sets  **LEVEL III** 7 sets  **REST** up to 2 minutes

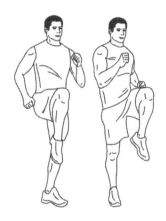

**20** high knees

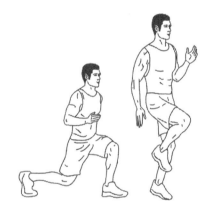

**20** lunge ste-ups

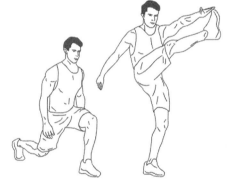

**20** lunge kicks

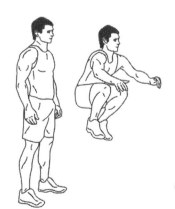

**10** jump knee tucks

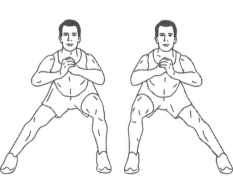

**10** side-to-side lunges

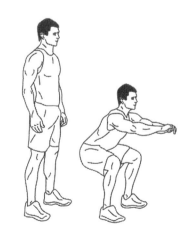

**10** squats

## 85 Push, squat, repeat

Sometimes what you want is to be able to simply do something simple. No overthinking the part, no role-play in your head. Nothing that will constantly challenge your coordination and force you to be mindful of your body every single moment of the workout. This is where this "Wash, Rinse and Repeat" cycle is perfect. You can set it up and let your body do its thing while your mind takes a figurative break for a while. So, choose your level and get ready to rock it.

**Focus: Strength & Tone**

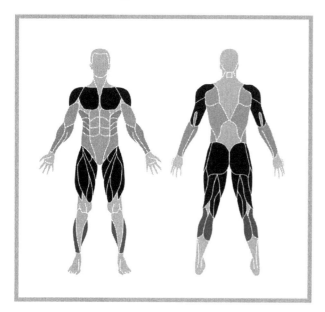

**LEVEL I** 3 sets
**LEVEL II** 5 sets
**LEVEL III** 7 sets
**REST** up to 2 minutes

# PUSH SQUAT REPEAT

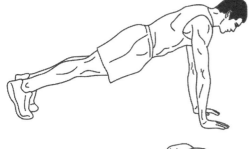

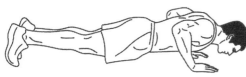

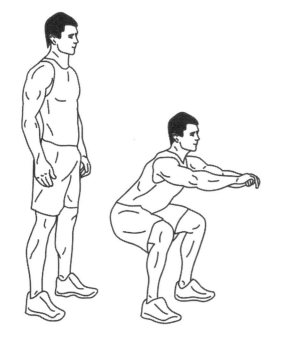

| | |
|---:|:---|
| **4 reps** | push-ups |
| **4 reps** | squats |
| **10 reps** | push-ups |
| **10 reps** | squats |
| **4 reps** | push-ups |
| **4 reps** | squats |
| **10 reps** | push-ups |
| **10 reps** | squats |
| | rest |

## 86 Quicksilver

Move faster without stressing your joints with the Quicksilver workout. It helps you develop muscle stability and mobility almost by stealth, its exercises are perfect for that indoor workout on days when you have a sofa handy.

Make it harder. When marching breathe out every time you raise your knees and slightly tense your lower abs, activating them.

**Focus: High Burn**

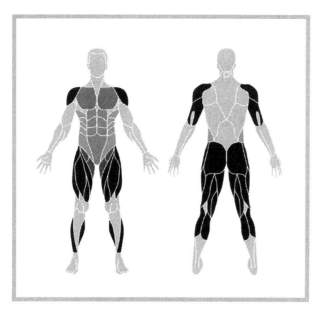

# QUICK SILVER

DAREBEE WORKOUT
© darebee.com
**LEVEL I** 3 sets
**LEVEL II** 5 sets
**LEVEL III** 7 sets
**REST** up to 2 minutes

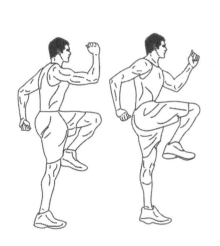

**20** march steps

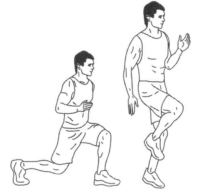

**20** lunge step-ups

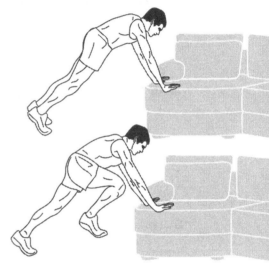

**20** incline slow climbers

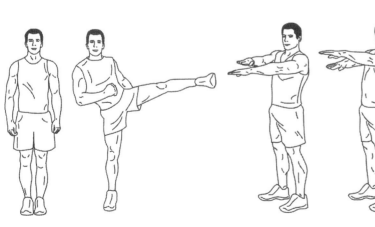

**10** side leg raises

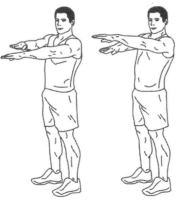

**10** arm scissors

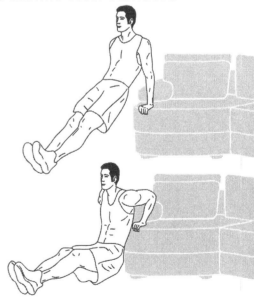

**10** tricep dips

## 87 Ranger

Rangers are known for stamina, strength, speed and agility and the Ranger workout takes you through each component in turn. You get to feel the heat building up under your skin and sense your muscles working, so you know that you are making gains. Rangers, of course, simply do not quit which is why you're doing this workout. We get it.

Make it harder: Bring your knees to waist height as you perform High Knees.

**Focus: High Burn, HIIT**

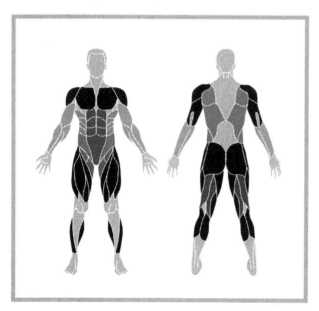

# RANGER

DAREBEE `HIIT` WORKOUT © darebee.com

**Level I** 5 rounds   **Level II** 10 rounds   **Level III** 15 rounds

1 minute rest between rounds

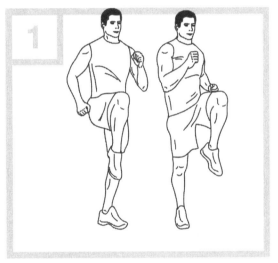

**20sec** high knees

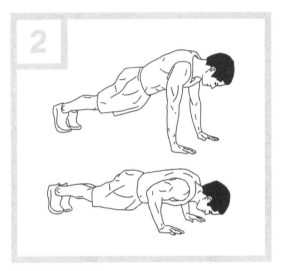

**20sec** push-ups

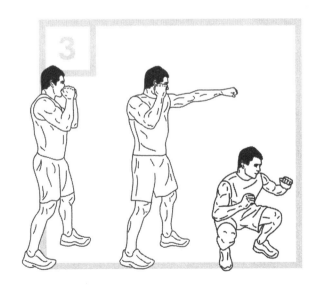

**20sec** jab + jab + cross + squat

## 88 Rebel

Rebels acknowledge no rules which means they have to be ready for anything. Our Rebel workout prepares you for almost anything. Its combination of static and ballistic exercises puts your body through its paces in a way that says "I am really preparing to break the rules".

**Focus: High Burn**

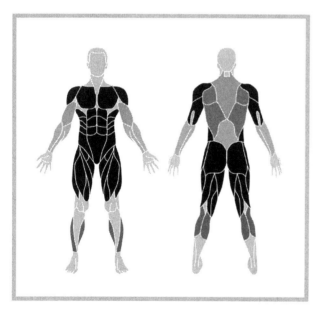

# REBEL

DAREBEE WORKOUT
© darebee.com
**LEVEL I** 3 sets
**LEVEL II** 5 sets
**LEVEL III** 7 sets
**REST** up to 2 minutes

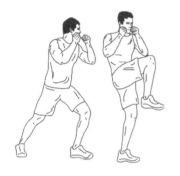 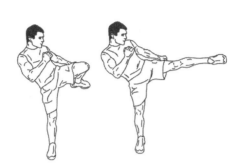 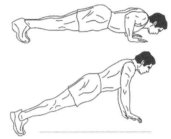

**40** knee strikes    **40** turning kicks    **10** power push-ups

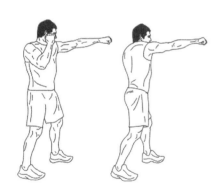 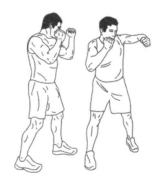 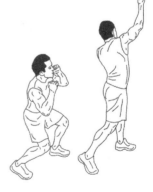

**20combos**  jab + jab + cross + hook + upper cut

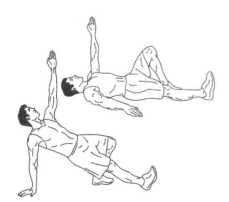 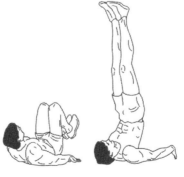 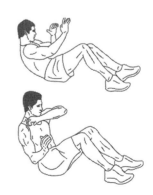

**10** get-ups    **10** butt-ups    **10** elbow strike sit-ups

## 89 Red Warrior

All warriors have the same things in common. Grit, perseverance. A high tolerance to failure. The willingness to keep on going whatever the odds and simply not give up. The Red Warrior workout is designed to help you find that warrior core within that allows you to overcome anything.

Tips When performing plank back kicks tense your lower abs, keeping your trunk immobile and working your glutes, hamstring and quads.

**Focus: Strength & Tone**

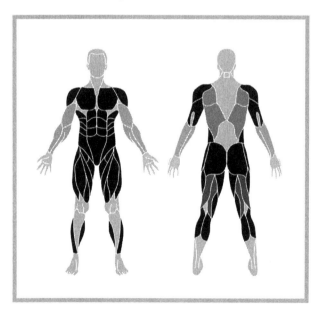

# RED WARRIOR

DAREBEE WORKOUT © darebee.com
**LEVEL I** 3 sets **LEVEL II** 5 sets **LEVEL III** 7 sets
**REST** up to 2 minutes

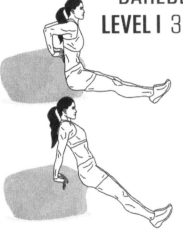 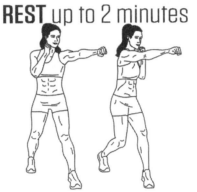 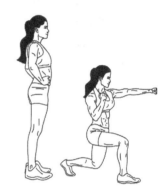

**20** tricep dips  **40** punches  **20** lunge punches

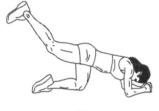
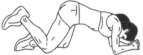 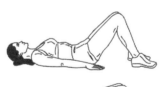
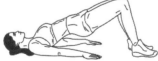 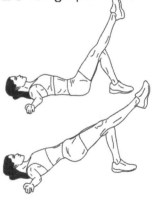

**10** plank back kicks  **10** bridges  **10** raised leg bridges

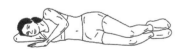
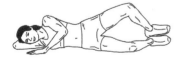 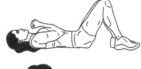
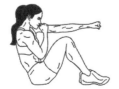 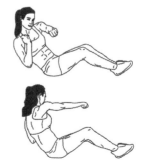

**10** clamshells  **10** sit-up punches  **10** sitting punches

# 90 Roaster

Getting your muscles to the point where you can practically feel the heat coming off them gives the sentence "going for the burn" an entirely new meaning altogether. The Roaster workout helps you attack some major muscle groups again and again from one exercise to another, varying the load, movement and intensity while still engaging the muscles. You will feel your body's temperature rise and you will feel the burn and after it's all over you should feel positively roasted.

**Focus: High Burn**

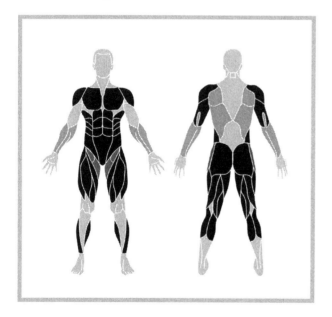

# THE ROASTER

DAREBEE WORKOUT © darebee.com

**LEVEL I** 3 sets  **LEVEL II** 5 sets  **LEVEL III** 7 sets  **REST** up to 2 minutes

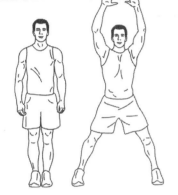

**20** jumping jacks

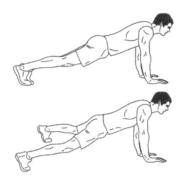

**2** plank jacks

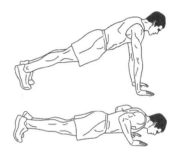

**2** push-ups (fast!)

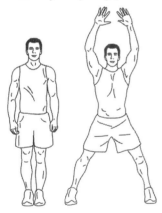

**20** jumping jacks

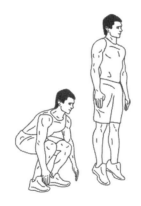

**2** jump squats

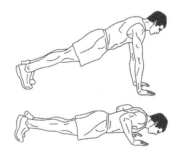

**2** push-ups (fast!)

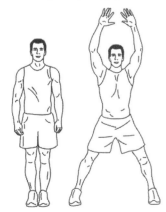

**20** jumping jacks

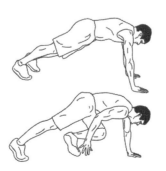

**2** climber taps

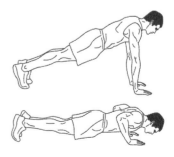

**2** push-ups (fast!)

## 91 Rogue

Rogues set their own rules which means they are self-sufficient, in control of their world. The Rogue workout builds strength where you need it so that you can make your body do what you command it to. What rules it then gets to play by is entirely up to you.

Make it harder. When performing jump squats clear the floor by at least a foot increasing the load on your quads, glutes and calves and maximizing the benefits of the exercise.

**Focus: High Burn**

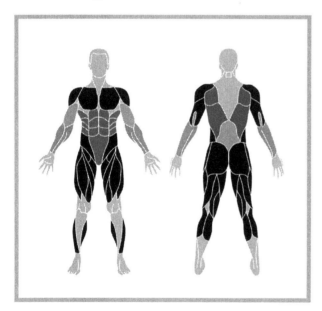

# ROGUE

DAREBEE WORKOUT © darebee.com

**LEVEL I** 3 sets   **LEVEL II** 5 sets   **LEVEL III** 7 sets

**REST** up to 2 minutes

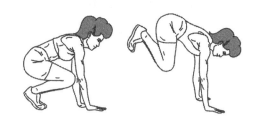

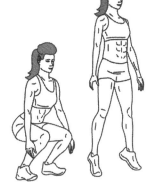

**20 combos:** hop heel click + floor tap heel click

**10** jump squats

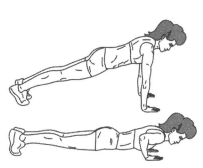

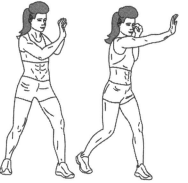

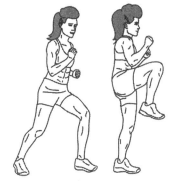

**10 combos:** push-up + palm strikes (each hand)

**20** knee strikes

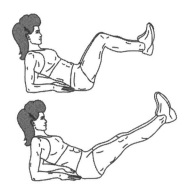

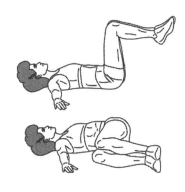

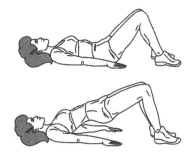

**10** crunch kicks

**10** half windshield wipers

**10** bridges

## 92 Run, you clever boy

Doctor Who fans will know that the moment you have to run you need to rely on limb speed and aerobic capacity. Well this workout helps you develop both.

Tips: This is a running work out so perform the high knees as high and as fast as possible and use the ground exercise to recover.

**Focus: High Burn**

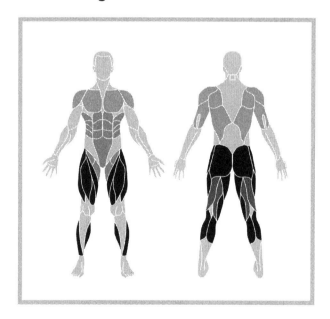

# RUN, YOU CLEVER BOY; AND REMEMBER

**DAREBEE WORKOUT** © darebee.com

**LEVEL I** 3 sets  **LEVEL II** 5 sets  **LEVEL III** 7 sets  **REST** up to 2 minutes

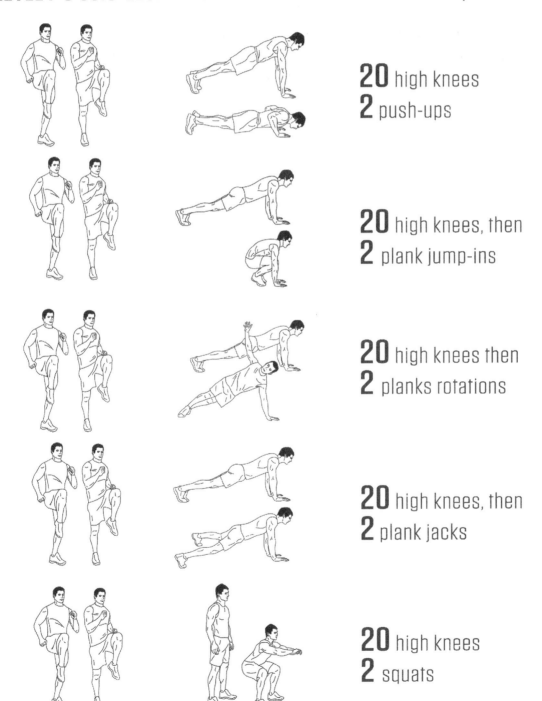

**20** high knees
**2** push-ups

**20** high knees, then
**2** plank jump-ins

**20** high knees then
**2** planks rotations

**20** high knees, then
**2** plank jacks

**20** high knees
**2** squats

## 93    Seated Yoga

If you have just three minutes in your day and a chair to sit on you can have a workout. Yoga is frequently underrated as a workout and yet a mini-break like that practiced whenever possible activates the muscles of the body, helps increase circulation and breathing and plays an incredible role in maintaining good health and the metabolic rate working properly.

**Focus: Stretching, Yoga**

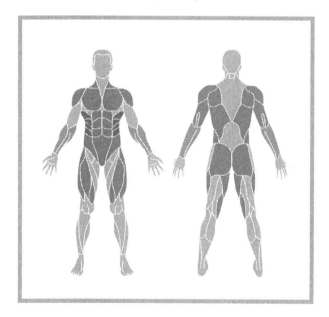

# 3-minute
# seated *Yoga*

DAREBEE WORKOUT
© darebee.com
30 seconds each

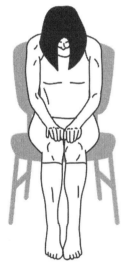

body fold

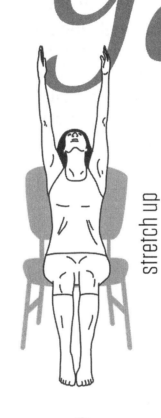

stretch up

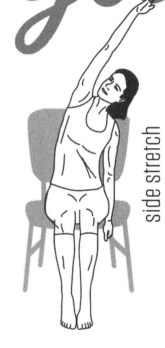

side stretch

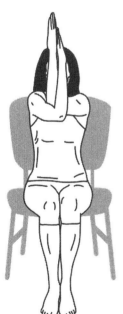

lotus twist

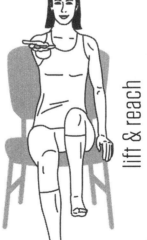

lift & reach

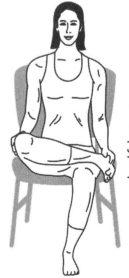

half lotus

## 94  Shieldmaiden

Shieldmaidens fought in battle and often led their own men. To match a hardened warrior, armed to the teeth and bristling with muscle you need more than just strength. You need fortitude, some killer tendon strength, agility and a core of steel, oh, and as much upper body strength as you can muster. The Shieldmaiden workout is designed to take you through your paces, give you a little of what you need and a lot of what you want (or is it the other way around?). Either way, you will definitely come out tougher at the other end of it.

**Focus: High Burn**

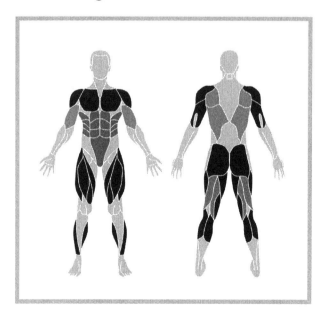

# shieldmaiden

DAREBEE WORKOUT © darebee.com

**LEVEL I** 3 sets  **LEVEL II** 5 sets  **LEVEL III** 7 sets  **REST** up to 2 minutes

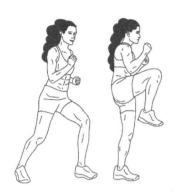

**20** knee strikes

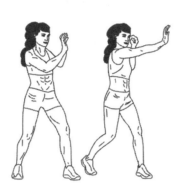

**20** palm strikes

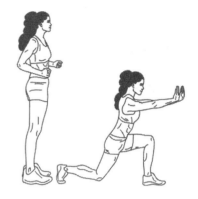

**20** lunge push strikes

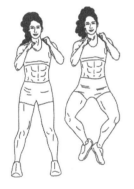

**10combos** hop heel click + palm strike

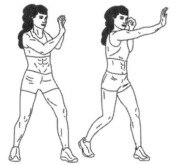

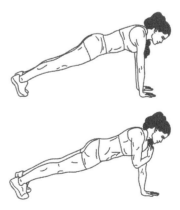

**10** push-ups

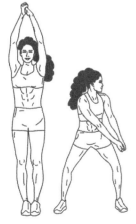

**20** cross chops

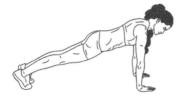

**20sec** plank hold

**20** shoulder taps

## 95 Shifter

Do shifters need to have great freedom of movement to physically morph from one form to another? We don't know for sure. But we do know that if you have the moves then you can walk the walk and talk the talk.

Tips: Practice the basic burpees in a controlled, flowing motion so that there is no break as you move from one position to the next. This allows for greater tendon strength as well as increased muscle density.

**Focus:  High Burn, HIIT**

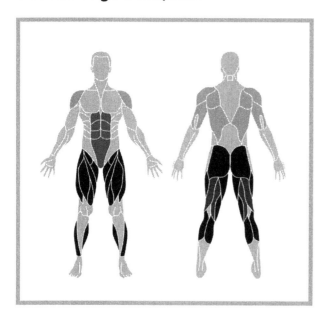

# SHIFTER

DAREBEE **HIIT** WORKOUT © darebee.com

**Level I** 5 rounds **Level II** 10 rounds **Level III** 15 rounds

1 minute rest between rounds

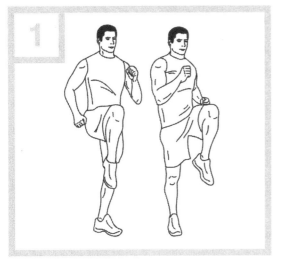

**20sec** high knees

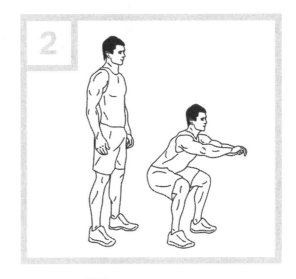

**20sec** squats

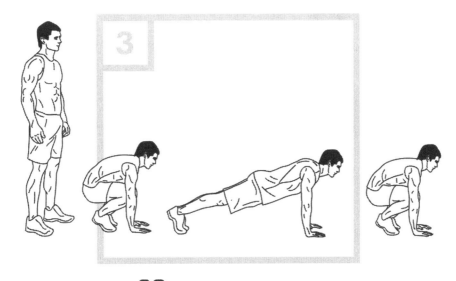

**20sec** basic burpees

# 96  Silver

The silver workout is a deceptively gentle set of exercises designed to get your body going without too much fanfare or undue pressure on muscle groups. This makes it one of those stealth mode workouts you can do when you're not sure you should be exercising or when you are in recuperative mode, or when simply you're stuck for a workout routine, do not want to wake the neighbours or advertise the fact you're working out. Plus, this is perfect for those just starting out on their journey to personal awesomeness.

**Focus: High Burn, HIIT**

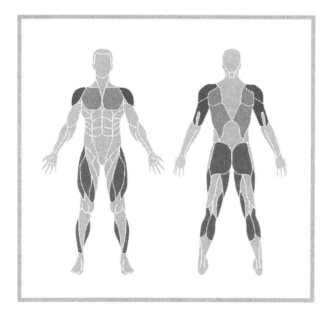

# SILVER

DAREBEE HIIT WORKOUT © darebee.com

**Level I** 5 rounds   **Level II** 10 rounds   **Level III** 15 rounds

1 minute rest between rounds

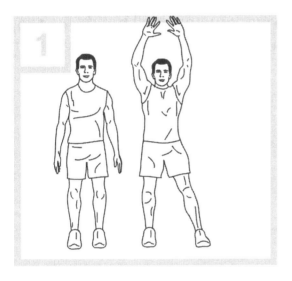

**20sec** step jacks

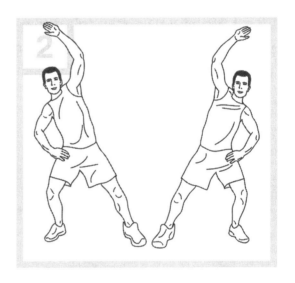

**20sec** step side jacks

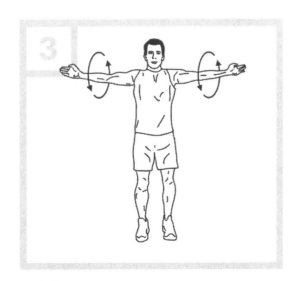

**20sec** raised arm rotations

## 97 Sofa Abs

At the end of a busy day, all you want is the chance to put work out of your mind, land on the sofa, turn the telly on and ... work your abs. The sofa's your gym. Your body is your equipment. This is the Sofa Abs workout. If you're on the sofa, it's time to work your abs.

Make it harder. You shouldn't. It's a sofa workout, after all but if you happen to have a pair of ankle weights lying around, now's the time to strap them on.

**Focus: Abs**

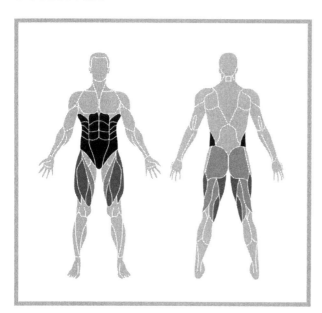

# sofa abs

DAREBEE WORKOUT © darebee.com

**LEVEL I** 3 sets  **LEVEL II** 4 sets  **LEVEL III** 5 sets  **REST** up to 2 minutes

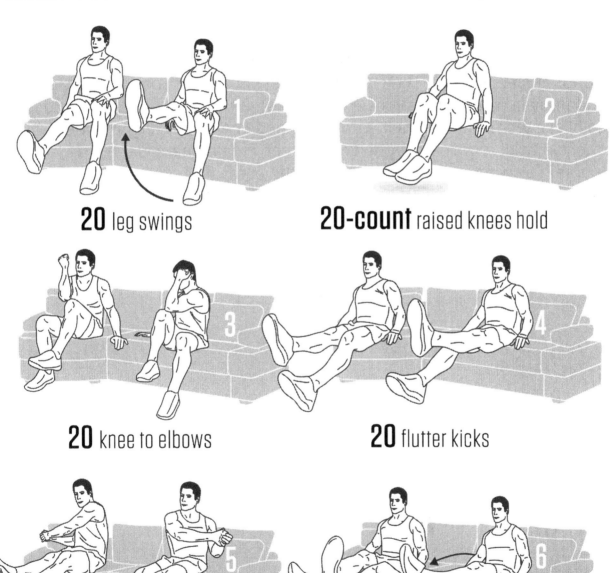

**20** leg swings

**20-count** raised knees hold

**20** knee to elbows

**20** flutter kicks

**10** raised legs twists

**10** scissors

## 98 Standing Abs

There is more than one way to train your abs. The ab wall is made up of four distinct muscle groups: Rectus Abdominis (the traditional six-pack you see in the movies and which every superhero sports) - it helps you move your lower and upper body, together. External Obliques - these are the muscles stretching over your ribs (the ones that really ache if you do a lot of push-ups, fast). They help you twist your body from side to side (and throw a punch or jump over obstacles). Internal Obliques - you do not really see them, but they help bring your body back into alignment every time you twist it in one direction or another. Finally there is the Transverse Abdominis - what we so popularly call "the core". These wrap around the spine and provide stability, keep us upright and make sure we don't get back pain from our upright posture. The standing abs workout targets all four muscle groups for a performance-enhancing experience.

**Focus: Abs**

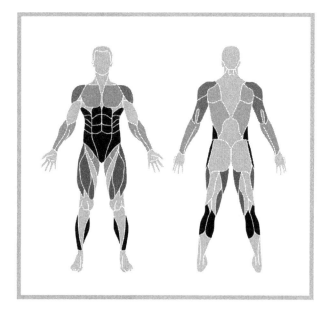

# standing abs

DAREBEE WORKOUT © darebee.com
**repeat 3 times** | up to 2 minute rest between sets

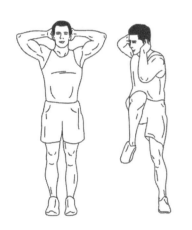

**20** knee-to-elbows

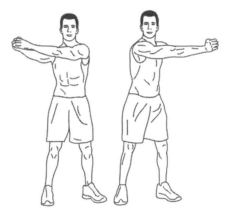

**20** side-to-side chops

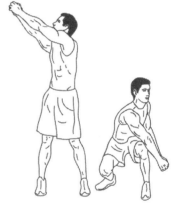

**10** cross chops

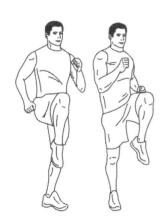

**20** high knees

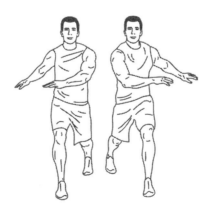

**20** twist jacks

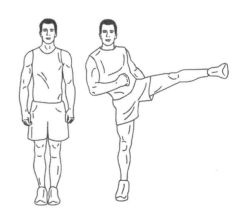

**10** side leg raises

## 99    Star Master

Good balance requires a strong core and great supporting muscle groups. The Star Master workout is designed to help you develop the kind of balance that marks exceptional athletic performance and the kind of badass muscle control that warrior-types achieve.

Instructions: Tap each point clockwise for 3 minutes then switch sides - and tap each point counterclockwise with the other leg for 3 minutes - 6 minutes in total.

**Focus: High Burn**

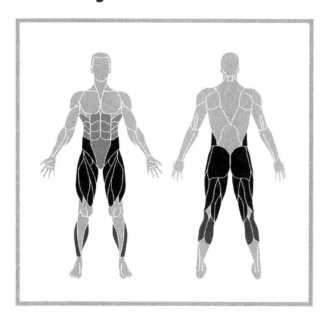

# Star Master

DAREBEE WORKOUT © darebee.com

Instructions: balance on one leg and tap with the other.

3 minutes right leg clockwise
3 minutes left leg counterclockwise
6 minutes in total

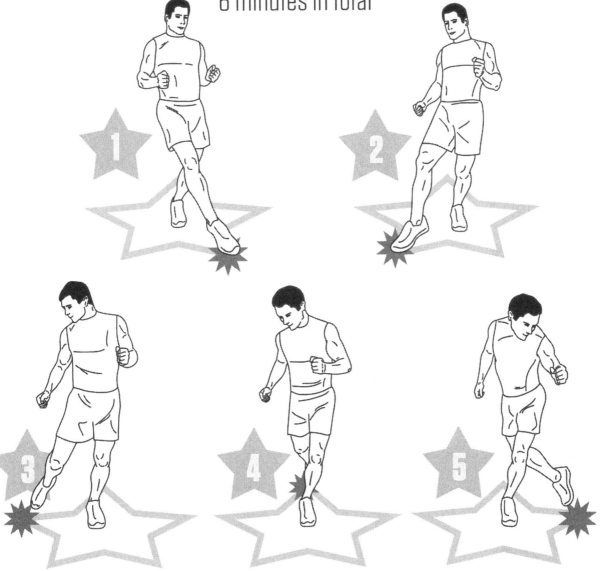

## 100 Swan

Ballet looks deceptively easy but anyone who has tried it knows it is exceptionally difficult requiring great balance, strength, flexibility and coordination, not to mention endurance. Ballet training is great for dancers, obviously, but it is also used by martial artists and boxers who need to move more creatively in very limited space. Try it and get to work muscles of your body you've never used properly, before.

**Focus: Strength & Tone**

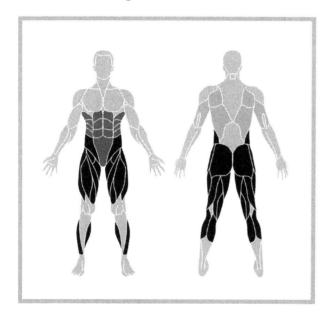

# Swan

DAREBEE WORKOUT © darebee.com

**LEVEL I** 3 sets **LEVEL II** 5 sets **LEVEL III** 7 sets **REST** up to 2 minutes

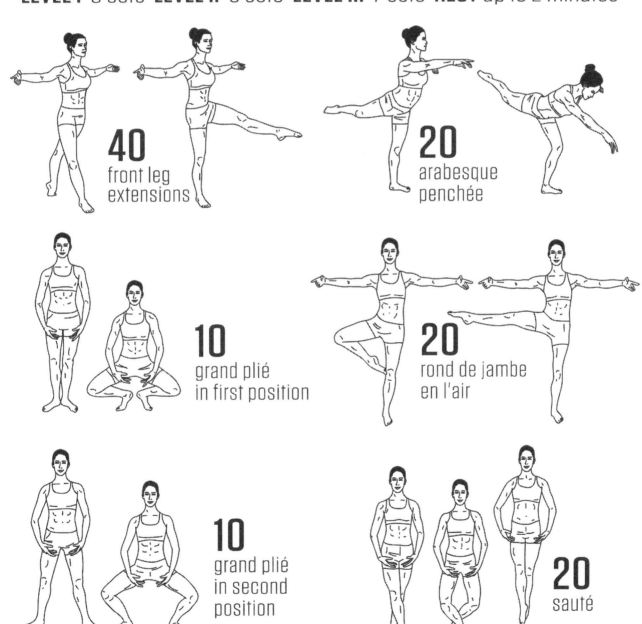

**40** front leg extensions

**20** arabesque penchée

**10** grand plié in first position

**20** rond de jambe en l'air

**10** grand plié in second position

**20** sauté